CLINICAL CHEMISTRY

KU-265-684

MADE EASY

Jeremy Hughes MA FRCPE PhD
Wellcome Trust Senior Research Fellow in Clinical Science and
Honorary Consultant Physician at the Royal Infirmary Edinburgh,
MRC Centre for Inflammation Research, The Queen's Medical
Research Institute, Edinburgh, UK

Ashley Jefferson MD MRCP
Clinical Associate Professor, Division of Nephrology, University of
Washington, Seattle, USA

Foreword by
John Iredale DM FRCP FMedSci
Professor of Medicine, University of Edinburgh

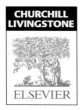

Edinburgh London New York Oxford Philadelphia St Louis Sydney Toronto 2008

CHURCHILL LIVINGSTONE
ELSEVIER

QY 90
A080922

CHURCHILL LIVINGSTONE
An imprint of Elsevier Limited

First published 2008

ISBN: 978-0-443-07197-3

International edition ISBN: 978-0-443-07196-6

British Library Cataloguing in Publication Data
A catalogue record for this book is available from the British Library

Library of Congress Cataloging in Publication Data
A catalog record for this book is available from the Library of Congress

Notice
Knowledge and best practice in this field are constantly changing. As new research and experience broaden our knowledge, changes in practice, treatment and drug therapy may become necessary or appropriate. Readers are advised to check the most current information provided (i) on procedures featured or (ii) by the manufacturer of each product to be administered, to verify the recommended dose or formula, the method and duration of administration, and contraindications. It is the responsibility of the practitioner, relying on their own experience and knowledge of the patient, to make diagnoses, to determine dosages and the best treatment for each individual patient, and to take all appropriate safety precautions. To the fullest extent of the law, neither the Publisher nor the Authors assume any liability for any injury and/or damage to persons or property arising out or related to any use of the material contained in this book.

The Publisher

Printed in China

Contents

Foreword

The functions of cells are governed by the laws of chemistry and physics, and biochemical reactions underlie the fundamental processes of life. For these reasons, it is no surprise that in many countries a high school chemistry qualification is a prerequisite for undergraduate admission to medical school. Medical students become exposed to biochemistry during their early training and many joke about the impenetrability of the subject. Indeed one classmate of mine, a witty songwriter, penned the classic 'Don't cry for me biochemistry, the truth is I never learnt you', to be sung to the tune of 'Don't cry for me Argentina', from the then hit Lloyd Webber musical 'Evita'. Of course, this levity disguises the fact that medical graduates invariably acquire a good working knowledge of biochemical process.

Having acquired a grounding in biochemistry, as clinical students and junior doctors we are then confronted with the challenge of assimilating that knowledge with the practice of medicine and exploiting it in clinical practice. Nowhere is that assimilation more direct than the field of clinical chemistry. However, the expanding content of undergraduate syllabuses means that the time and opportunity to make this synthesis is becoming eroded. Moreover, the integration of pre-clinical biochemistry with the approach to clinical problems is not always straightforward. For example, understanding the Henderson–Hasselbalch equation and the principles underlying pH balance and buffering may seem straightforward in abstract, but grouping the patterns of changes in pH and accompanying alterations in the PO_2 and PCO_2 in the blood gases of a breathless patient can seem daunting to the medical student and junior doctor. The approach to clinical chemistry in real clinical situations requires knowledge, experience and an integrated and clinically relevant model. It is precisely this integrated model which Jeremy Hughes and Ashley Jefferson have brought together in this text.

The use of appropriate clinical context throughout the book illustrates how clinical chemistry tests can be deployed to rapidly obtain information critical for the management of sick patients. This area of medicine is now of essential importance given the changes in the process of care delivery in hospitals. Junior doctors are frequently called to see sick patients with whom they are unfamiliar, and for whom a rapid appraisal of clinical need and diagnosis will be required. The armamentarium of clinical chemistry tests is invaluable in this setting – frequently simple investigations, such as blood gas measurements, can rapidly provide information essential to diagnosis and management. Far from being a setting neglected by the authors, clear and concise guidance to the use and interpretation of tests in the emergency setting is a particular strength of this volume. An additional area of focus is the role of drugs in influencing the results of clinical chemistry tests and as possible causes of abnormalities in routine tests undertaken in both the community and hospital settings. With the increasing number of elderly patients who are all too frequently exposed to polypharmacy, this area also will assume a greater and greater importance in the diagnosis and effective management of our patient population.

This concise and highly readable text provides exactly the information that senior clinical students and junior doctors need to request, arrange and interpret clinical chemistry tests effectively, and in so doing enhance clinical care. It is the kind of book I wish had been available when I was a student and should be valuable to trainees across all specialities. There is no longer any excuse for biochemistry and clinical chemistry to be a neglected or 'tearful' partner in the curriculum.

John Iredale
Edinburgh 2007

Preface

Clinicians are unable to provide adequate medical care in isolation. They are dependent upon numerous laboratory disciplines to assist in the management of patients with varied medical problems. Departments of Clinical Chemistry and related departments such as Microbiology and Clinical Immunology play a very important role in patient care. They provide critically important information that may be either diagnostic, as in the levels of cardiac enzymes, or facilitate the accurate monitoring of conditions such as systemic inflammation or hepatic failure. Although many of these tests may be interpreted in isolation, it is usually important to examine any 'trends' that are evident, e.g. deterioration in renal function, overall control of diabetes mellitus.

It is imperative to realise that the use of simple clinical acumen and skill is a critically important facet of patient care. It is always inadequate to investigate a patient by simply 'ordering a few tests'. Although there is unquestionably a role for routine screening tests in certain patient populations, it is useful to request and interpret pertinent investigations in the clinical context of the individual patient. Indeed, significant errors in clinical management may ensue if data derived from laboratory investigations are acted upon without an adequate clinical assessment of the patient.

Junior clinical staff are typically the first point of contact for ward staff who are concerned about the condition of inpatients during the night or at the weekend. Often, junior doctors will be required to assess and treat patients 'out of hours', despite the fact that they may not be directly involved in their routine medical care. The key to success in these circumstances is:

1. Get to grips with the acute problem, pertinent medical background and current drug treatment.
2. Examine the patient briefly with particular emphasis upon the relevant physiological system.
3. If the diagnosis is not apparent then make a differential diagnosis and institute tests that will enable you to make a definitive diagnosis. This may include clinical chemistry, haematological, radiological and cardiological investigations.
4. Reconsider the clinical situation when the results of investigations become available and integrate all of the available data. It may well be necessary to institute appropriate therapy at this point.

5. If the situation is problematical then seek the advice of a senior colleague at an early stage.

In addition, it is not uncommon for junior medical staff to be contacted regarding an 'abnormal test result' that has come back. This book has been written with the above practical tips in mind and the integration of clinical and laboratory data emphasised. It is our hope that this book will help the reader develop and hone the skills necessary to deal effectively with patients in diverse circumstances.

2008 Edinburgh, JH
Seattle, AJ

CHAPTER 1

Sodium and water balance

Introduction

Abnormalities of sodium and water balance are the commonest fluid and electrolyte abnormalities in clinical medicine. Both hyponatraemia and hypernatraemia may have serious consequences but, as will be outlined in this chapter, the treatment of these conditions is not without risk.

> It is important to recognise that sodium balance and water balance are controlled separately. Abnormalities in sodium balance lead to changes in the extracellular volume (volume depletion or volume overload), whereas abnormalities in water balance lead to changes in the serum sodium concentration (hyponatraemia or hypernatraemia).

Distribution

Some 60% of the weight of an adult male (50% in females) is water and termed the total body water (TBW). This is distributed between the intracellular fluid (ICF) and the extracellular fluid (ECF). The ECF is further divided into interstitial fluid and plasma (Fig. 1.1). As water

ICF ($^2/_3$ TBW)		ECF ($^1/_3$ TBW)	
		Interstitial fluid	Plasma
28 L		11 L	3 L
Na$^+$	10	Na$^+$	140
K$^+$	150	K$^+$	4.5
Cl$^-$	4	Cl$^-$	104
HCO$_3^-$	12	HCO$_3^-$	24
PO$_4^{3-}$	140	PO$_4^{3-}$	1

Figure 1.1 Composition of water and electrolytes in body compartments of a 70-kg man. Data expressed as concentrations (mmol/L). Note that sodium is the major extracellular fluid cation and potassium the major intracellular fluid cation.

can move freely across cell membranes, the size of the ICF and ECF is determined by the number of osmotically active particles in each of these spaces. There are approximately twice as many osmoles in the ICF (mostly potassium and organic phosphates) as in the ECF (mostly sodium, the accompanying anions chloride and bicarbonate together with albumin), and therefore two-thirds of TBW is in the ICF and one-third is in the ECF. Sodium is maintained predominantly in the ECF by the action of the Na–K-ATPase pump in cell membranes.

Control of sodium balance

The average daily Western diet contains 150–200 mmol of sodium which must be excreted to avoid volume overload. The kidneys are primarily responsible for excreting the daily sodium load. With a normal glomerular filtration rate (GFR) of 180 L per day, approximately 25 000 mmol of sodium are filtered at the glomerulus, with less than 1% of this being excreted in the urine (approx. 150 mmol/d). The majority of filtered sodium is reabsorbed along the nephrons, with the majority of sodium being reabsorbed in the proximal tubule (Fig. 1.2).

Abnormalities of sodium balance lead to volume depletion or volume expansion.

Volume depletion (decreased total body sodium)

Volume depletion is sensed by arterial (carotid) and venous baroreceptors leading to activation of angiotensin II, aldosterone and the

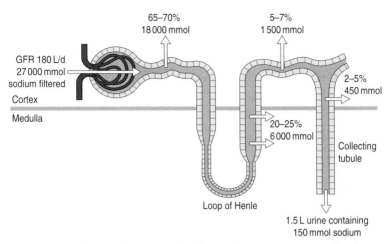

Figure 1.2 Sodium reabsorption along the nephron. Large amounts of sodium are filtered at the glomeruli daily, with the majority of filtered sodium being reabsorbed.

sympathetic nervous system, and decreased activity of natriuretic peptides. In this setting, the kidneys will retain filtered sodium and typically excrete urine with a sodium concentration of less than 10 mmol/L.

Volume overload (increased total body sodium)

Conversely, in the setting of an increased sodium load (volume overload), excess sodium can be excreted in the urine due to an increased GFR (pressure natriuresis), increased natriuretic peptides and inhibition of the renin–angiotensin system and aldosterone.

Control of water balance

Water balance is controlled primarily by thirst and the production of either a dilute or concentrated urine. Urinary concentration is under the control of antidiuretic hormone (ADH). ADH is a nine-amino-acid peptide secreted by the posterior lobe of the pituitary gland. ADH acts on the cells of the medullary collecting duct and stimulates the insertion of aquaporin 2 water channels into the luminal membrane of the epithelial cells. This allows the reabsorption of water from the tubular lumen into the hypertonic medulla which is established by the countercurrent system (Fig. 1.3).

Abnormalities of water balance lead to hyponatraemia or hypernatraemia.

Water excess (hyponatraemia)

In this setting thirst is inhibited, the plasma osmolality falls, and this suppresses the release of ADH. The absence of ADH reduces the

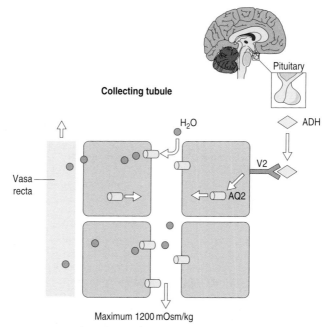

Figure 1.3 Action of antidiuretic hormone (ADH). ADH is produced by the hypothalamus and stored in the pituitary gland. The binding of ADH to the V2 receptors on principal cells in the medullar, collecting duct results in the insertion of aquaporin 2 (AQ2) water channels into the luminal membrane. This allows the reabsorption of water from the ultrafiltrate with a resultant increase in the concentration of the urine.

Table 1.1 Causes of antidiuretic hormone release

Hyperosmolality	Hypernatraemia
	Hyperglycaemia
Decreased effective arterial blood volume	Volume depletion
	Severe cardiac failure
	Liver failure
Stress	Postoperative
	Nausea
	Pain

permeability of the collecting ducts to water, allowing the passage of a dilute urine (minimum urinary osmolality 25–50 mOsm/kg). This effectively excretes the excess water with a resultant increase in the serum sodium level.

Water depletion (hypernatraemia)

By contrast, in setting of water depletion (hypernatraemia), the plasma osmolality becomes raised and stimulates ADH release. This results in the production of urine that is concentrated (maximal 1200 mOsm/kg) and the subsequent retention of water.

It should be noted that ADH can be stimulated by factors other than hypertonicity (Table 1.1). Volume depletion stimulates ADH synthesis, and hyponatraemia is typically found in settings of volume depletion or a decreased effective arterial blood volume (e.g. heart failure, liver disease). The restoration of plasma volume takes precedence over osmolality and ADH is stimulated in volume depletion despite the presence of hypo-osmolality.

When should I check sodium level?

The measurement of serum sodium together with other electrolytes is commonly performed in 'everyday' clinical practice, e.g. preoperative bloods, outpatient clinics. However, there are indications for specifically checking the serum sodium. These include:

- Seriously ill patients including those who are unconscious or obtunded
- Patients with significant cardiac, renal or liver disease

- Patients receiving intravenous fluids or parenteral nutrition
- Patients receiving drugs that may affect serum sodium levels including diuretics (a very common cause of hyponatraemia)
- Patients with uncontrolled diabetes mellitus
- Patients with polyuria or polydipsia.

What do I do with the result?

In the majority of instances, an abnormal sodium level will not require urgent action. Indeed, the over-enthusiastic treatment of hyponatraemia or hypernatraemia may be dangerous. However, the clinician should look for 'trends', as it may well be possible to adjust therapy to *prevent* the development of severe hyponatraemia or hypernatraemia (e.g. fluid restriction, a reduction in diuretic dosage or adjustment of intravenous fluid therapy). If the sodium level is below 120 mmol/L or greater than 160 mmol/L, then active treatment should be considered.

Hyponatraemia (serum Na <135 mmol/L)

Hyponatraemia is best considered an abnormality of water balance representing an excess of water relative to sodium. Although sodium loss can cause hyponatraemia, this rarely happens in excess of water loss and therefore does not cause hyponatraemia directly. Instead, sodium loss causes ECF depletion with subsequent volume-mediated activation of ADH leading to an impairment of electrolyte free water (EFW) excretion.

Two factors are required to develop hyponatraemia

1. *A source of electrolyte free water* (usually oral or intravenous (i.v.) fluids, rarely EFW generation from hypertonic urine). It should be noted that the ingestion of excess free water alone (psychogenic polydipsia) rarely causes hyponatraemia in the absence of impaired urinary dilution.
2. *An impaired ability of the kidneys to excrete dilute urine.* This impaired ability may be due to:
   (a) defective ADH action (this the commonest cause; see Table 1.1)
   (b) a low urine output which may result from (i) severe renal failure e.g. GFR <10 mL/min or (ii) a markedly decreased urine solute load. There is a minimum level to which the kidneys can dilute the urine ($\sim$50 mOsm/kg) and this may be limited by a reduction

in the daily solute load, e.g. tea and toast diet in the elderly or beer potomania.

Learning point

Hyponatraemia is often asymptomatic. A decreased sodium intake alone is not a common cause of hyponatraemia and persistent hyponatraemia is often found in patients with defective homeostatic mechanisms.

Assessment of the patient

1. *Is this pseudohyponatraemia?* This may be found in patients with severe hypertriglyceridaemia or severe paraproteinaemia. It is very rare and is detected by a normal serum osmolality despite hyponatraemia.
2. *Is the hyponatraemia acute (<48 h) or chronic?* This is a critical question as inappropriate treatment of hyponatraemia may be as dangerous as the hyponatraemia itself.
3. (i) *Acute hyponatraemia (<48 h).* The main risk is acute cerebral oedema secondary to water moving into brain cells. The treatment of acute hyponatraemia may need to be aggressive.
   (ii) *Chronic hyponatraemia (>48 h).* The main risk is overly aggressive therapy as rapid changes in plasma sodium levels may result in major neurological consequences (central pontine myelinolysis). The aim of treatment is to increase the plasma sodium level slowly.
4. Does the patient exhibit any acute neurological disturbance, such as seizures or confusion? Symptomatic hyponatraemia needs rapid treatment, generally with hypertonic saline.
5. *What is the volume status of the patient?* This assessment is the key to determining the underlying cause of the hyponatraemia and choosing the appropriate therapy.
6. *What is the source of the EFW?* This is the primary diagnostic question in patients with acute hyponatraemia. It is important to check i.v. fluids, TPN or enteral feeds as well as oral fluid intake. It is not uncommon for inappropriate prescribing of hypotonic fluids to be a factor in the development of hyponatraemia.
7. *Why are the kidneys not able to excrete the excess EFW?* This is the primary diagnostic question in patients with chronic hyponatraemia. Is it usually due to ADH secretion (see Table 1.1).

Laboratory tests

The laboratory tests required to assess hyponatraemia include serum osmolality, urine osmolality and urine sodium.

1. *Plasma osmolality* – this should be hypotonic (<280 mOsm/kg). Isotonic plasma (280–295 mOsm/kg) suggests pseudohyponatraemia, and hypertonic plasma (>295 mOsm/kg) suggests hyperglycaemia or rarely mannitol treatment.
2. *Urine osmolality* – this is typically raised (>100 mOsm/kg), confirming impaired renal excretion of EFW. Rarely the urine osmolality is low (<100 mOsm/kg), implying excess water intake.
3. *Urine sodium* – a low urine sodium level (<20 mmol/L) may suggest volume depletion which increases ADH release. It should be noted that there is a decreased effective arterial blood volume in oedematous states such as cardiac failure, liver failure and nephrotic syndrome. This results in both ADH release and impaired renal perfusion with a low urine sodium concentration.

Symptoms and signs

Clinical features are typically related to the central nervous system (CNS) and relate to both the degree of hyponatraemia and the rate of decline. Acute hyponatraemia leads to swelling of the brain cells, termed cerebral oedema. This may result in confusion, seizures, coma and tonsillar herniation in severe cases. Most patients with seizures and coma have serum sodium levels <120 mmol/L. By contrast, patients with chronic hyponatraemia are often asymptomatic or present with mild confusion or nausea. In these patients cerebral adaptation has occurred and the brain cells have excreted intracellular osmoles to limit cell swelling. In this setting, the over-rapid correction of chronic hyponatraemia may produce profound neurological abnormalities.

Differential diagnosis of hyponatraemia

This can be determined from the algorithm Figure 1.4. It is, however, important to note that several factors are often present in the same patient, e.g. thiazide diuretic use in an elderly patient with poor solute intake and mild chronic renal failure, with the latter two factors reducing the ability to dilute the urine maximally.

Hyperglycaemia

This is a common cause of hyponatraemia. Hyperglycaemia increases the serum osmolality and results in the movement of water from the

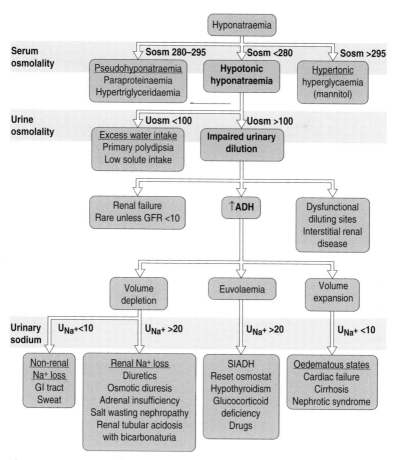

Figure 1.4 Causes of hyponatraemia.

ICF to the ECF in order to restore osmotic equilibrium. The serum sodium should fall by 3 mmol/L for every 10-mmol/L increase in blood glucose concentration. Urea and ethanol also raise the serum osmolality but move rapidly across cell membranes and are thus ineffective osmoles and do not alter the serum sodium level.

Pseudohyponatraemia

Sodium is distributed in the aqueous phase of plasma ($\sim$93% of plasma volume), but the expressed sodium concentration is based upon the total volume of plasma analysed. Rarely, a marked hypertriglycerid-aemia (>10–15 mmol/L) or severe paraproteinaemia (>100 g/L) may increase the non-aqueous phase and result in pseudohyponatraemia. The serum osmolality is normal in this setting.

Artefactual hyponatraemia

Artefactual hyponatraemia may occur when the blood sample is taken from a 'drip arm', i.e. there is an intravenous infusion of 5% dextrose or 'dextrose/saline' running into the arm when the blood sample is collected.

Iatrogenic

This is a very common cause of hyponatraemia in hospitalised patients due to inappropriate intravenous fluids. In the postoperative setting, there is often ADH release secondary to pain and stress, and excess 5% dextrose may result in hyponatraemia. It should be remembered that hospitalised patients often have additional sources of EFW, including oral fluids, parenteral nutrition or ice chips.

Polydipsia

Excess water intake alone is rarely the sole cause of hyponatraemia as normal kidneys can excrete close to 15–20 L of EFW per day. Some psychiatric patients may drink these very large amounts. In this setting the urine osmolality will be very low (<100 mOsm/kg). More commonly a large water intake contributes to the hyponatraemia that develops in the presence of impaired free water excretion, e.g. in the presence of ADH.

Diuretics and other drugs

Thiazide diuretics commonly cause hypovolaemic hyponatraemia due to volume depletion-mediated activation of ADH and ongoing EFW ingestion. Loop diuretics rarely cause this effect as the blockade of Na^+ reabsorption in the loop of Henle interferes with the maintenance of medullary hypertonicity, which impairs the action of ADH.

Other drugs associated with hyponatraemia are shown in Table 1.2.

Table 1.2 Drugs associated with hyponatraemia

Mechanism	Drug
ADH analogues	Vasopressin
	Desmopressin (DDAVP)
	Oxytocin
Stimulation of ADH release	Carbamazepine
	Chlorpropamide
	Antidepressants[a]
	Antipsychotic agents[a]
	Vincristine/vinblastine
	Narcotics
	Clofibrate
	Ifosfamide
Enhanced ADH renal effect	NSAIDs
	Chlorpropamide
	Cyclophosphamide

[a]Mechanism unknown for several of these agents. ADH, antidiuretic hormone; NSAIDs, non-steroidal anti-inflammatory drugs.

Syndrome of inappropriate ADH (SIADH)

Diagnostic criteria for SIADH

1. Hyponatraemia (<135 mmol/L)
2. Decreased serum osmolality (<270 mOsm/kg)
3. Urine sodium >20 mmol/L
4. Inappropriate urine concentration (urine osmolality >100 mOsm/kg)
5. Exclusion of renal failure and endocrine dysfunction

This is a common cause of hyponatraemia but is a diagnosis of exclusion. It is a disorder of osmoregulation where hypotonicity fails adequately to suppress the production of ADH. The causes of SIADH are categorised as pulmonary, neurological (CNS) or carcinoma (Table 1.3).

SIADH is diagnosed when hyponatraemia is present with evidence of ADH action (urine osmolality >100 mOsm/kg) and when other

Table 1.3 Causes of SIADH

Carcinomas	Pulmonary	Central nervous system
Bronchogenic	Pneumonia (viral/	Encephalitis (viral/bacterial)
Gastrointestinal	bacterial)	Meningitis (viral/bacterial/TB/
Bladder	Tuberculosis	fungal)
Prostate	Pulmonary abscess	Brain tumours
Pancreas	Aspergillosis	Brain abscess
	Mesothelioma	Cerebral haemorrhage

causes for ADH action have been excluded (hypovolaemia, oedematous states, endocrine dysfunction such as adrenal insufficiency and hypothyroidism, renal impairment or drugs). The urine sodium concentration is not reduced (>20 mmol/L), but reflects the daily sodium intake.

Management

Never treat a sodium concentration in isolation. Clinically important consequences often depend on *the rate of change of serum sodium levels* and not the absolute value.

Treatment of acute symptomatic hyponatraemia is a medical emergency. Treatment of chronic asymptomatic hyponatraemia must be cautious as over-aggressive therapy can have serious consequences. The treatment of hyponatraemia is related to both the underlying cause and the clinical severity. If symptoms are present (seizures, coma), this is a medical emergency. The underlying cause of the hyponatraemia must also be treated, e.g. pneumonia, tumour, etc.

Acute symptomatic hyponatraemia (<48 h)

Hyponatraemia complicated by symptomatic cerebral oedema should be treated rapidly. The correction rate should be 1–2 mmol/L/h over the first 3–4 h with a maximum correction of 12 mmol/L/24 h.

This condition typically arises in the postoperative setting in patients who have received excessive hypotonic intravenous fluids. It may also be seen in acute water intoxication (e.g. ecstasy use, psychogenic polydipsia). The main risk is cerebral oedema with potentially devastating neurological injury. For unclear reasons the neurological complications appear more common in women. Treatment guidelines include water restriction and:

1. Intravenous administration of hypertonic 3% saline (1–2 mL per kg bodyweight per h), which may be combined with furosemide to prevent sodium overload and increase EFW excretion.
2. If patients are severely obtunded or have seizures, the hypertonic saline may be administered at an increased rate (4–6 mL/kg/h) for a 2–3-h period to improve symptoms.

The goal is to raise the serum sodium level by 1–2 mmol/h over the first 3–4 h, but with a maximum increase of 12 mmol in 24 h. Vigilant monitoring (at least 2-hourly) is clearly mandatory during this acute stage. The saline used must be hypertonic to urine, otherwise the renal generation of EFW may occur and this will exacerbate the hyponatraemia.

Volume depletion

Patients with hyponatraemia secondary to volume depletion typically respond to isotonic normal saline, as correction of the volume depletion will remove the stimulus for ADH release and permit renal excretion of a maximally dilute urine. Great care must be taken as the rapid renal excretion of the excess water may correct the serum sodium level too quickly.

Chronic hyponatraemia (>48 h)

Over-rapid correction of serum Na^+ concentration in patients with chronic hyponatraemia can precipitate central pontine myelinolysis. The correction rate should be less than 1 mmol/L/h, with a maximum of 10–12 mmol/L over a 24-h period.

In patients with chronic hyponatraemia (>48 h) some cerebral adaptation has occurred and these patients are at risk of a demyelinating syndrome associated with flaccid paraplegia, dysarthria and dysphagia (central pontine myelinolysis) if the sodium is corrected too quickly.

Recommended therapeutic strategies include:

1. water restriction
2. increased salt intake with furosemide to promote renal EFW excretion
3. administration of drugs to antagonise the action of ADH (e.g. demeclocycline, conivaptan).

However, if the patient is symptomatic with seizures or a decreased level of consciousness then the initial treatment should be more rapid and aim to raise the serum sodium level by 1–2 mmol/L/h over the first 3–4 h.

Hypernatraemia (serum Na >145 mmol/L)

This represents a decrease in water relative to sodium, and is almost always due to a problem with water balance. Rarely, excess sodium intake causes hypernatraemia (e.g. iatrogenic, drinking sea water) when it is associated with a marked increase in ECF volume. It should be noted that hypernatraemia will not develop unless there is an impaired thirst mechanism or difficulties with access to water (hospitalised patients, infants and the elderly).

Symptoms and signs

Thirst is the predominant symptom of hypernatraemia. The serum hypertonicity promotes water movement from ICF to ECF, and results in cell shrinkage. CNS symptoms such as confusion or coma may occur if the hypernatraemia is severe (typically approaching 160 mmol/L). Marked brain cell shrinkage increases the risk of cerebral haemorrhage. It should be noted that patients with diabetes insipidus usually have a normal serum sodium level due to marked polydipsia compensating for the polyuria, but the sodium level may rise rapidly if they become unable to maintain their fluid intake, e.g. if vomiting.

Clinical assessment

1. *Is the ECF volume expanded?* Check for the presence of peripheral oedema, hypertension, cardiac failure, pulmonary oedema or a change in the patient's weight as this typically reflects a change in fluid status. Hypernatraemia is typically associated with a decreased bodyweight secondary to water loss. Although rare, the weight is increased with an expanded ECF volume in the setting of a significant gain of total body sodium.
2. *What is the source of the water loss?* Are there high insensible losses, e.g. fever, ventilation, excess sweating. Other causes include diarrhoea and high urinary losses secondary to polyuria, e.g. the recovery phase of acute tubular necrosis or glycosuria in poorly controlled diabetes.
3. *Why has there not been a compensatory increase in water intake?* Is the patient thirsty? A small increase in plasma tonicity should lead to

marked thirst, and the absence of thirst suggests a CNS lesion or altered mental status.

4. *Is the patient polyuric?* This may be due to an osmotic diuresis (urine osmolality 400–500 mOsm/kg) or a water diuresis (<150 mOsm/kg).

Laboratory results

The urine osmolality helps to differentiate between the three major causes of hypernatraemia: diabetes insipidus, osmotic diuresis (usually glucose) and the inadequate replacement of non-renal EFW loss. Serum hypertonicity stimulates ADH release such that the urine osmolality should be markedly increased (800–1200 mOsm/kg). A low urine osmolality suggests ADH deficiency secondary to reduced production (central diabetes insipidus) or a diminished renal responsiveness to ADH (nephrogenic diabetes insipidus).

Differential diagnosis

This can be determined from the algorithm in Figure 1.5.

Non-renal water loss

This typically occurs in the hospitalised patient or nursing home resident. Insensible losses (respiratory tract and sweat) are hypotonic and, if not replaced with adequate water, will lead to hypernatraemia. Gastrointestinal losses (diarrhoea) are also typically hypotonic (80–200 mOsm/kg) and may exacerbate EFW loss. Patients with diarrhoea often have a significant sodium loss in addition to the relatively greater water loss, and this is reflected by additional evidence of volume depletion on examination. When faced with non-renal water loss, the normal kidneys are able to produce a low volume of a urine with a high osmolality.

Osmotic diuresis

In this setting the urine osmolality is typically about 500 mOsm/kg and the urine contains close to 50 mmol/L Na^+ and 25–50 mmol/L K^+. The diagnosis should be suspected in patients with a high urine volume and a high urine osmolality. This results in a high osmole excretion rate (normal 600–900 mOsm per day). The most common cause is glycosuria secondary to hyperglycaemia. Occasionally a high urea excretion rate may cause urine water loss in excess of sodium, and this may be present in patients who are catabolic, receiving high protein feeding or recovering from acute renal failure.

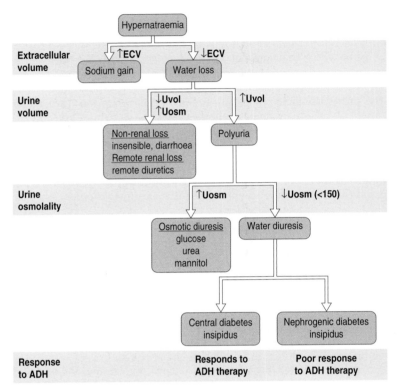

Figure 1.5 Causes of hypernatraemia.

Diabetes insipidus

Diabetes insipidus is characterised by the inability of the kidneys to concentrate the urine, resulting in polyuria. The patient typically has intense thirst and polydipsia. Although hypernatraemia will develop if water intake is insufficient, patients are often able to maintain the serum sodium level in the normal range by drinking large amounts of water (sometimes >10 L per day).

Diabetes insipidus is divided into

1. *Central diabetes insipidus.* This condition results from a deficiency of ADH and is caused by lesions to the hypothalamus or pituitary (Table 1.4). The onset of polyuria is often abrupt. Serum ADH levels are low and the urine osmolality is often markedly low (50–100 mOsm/kg).
2. *Nephrogenic diabetes insipidus.* This condition results from an abnormal renal response to ADH (see Table 1.4). Serum ADH levels are increased but the urine osmolality remains low (often 50–250 mOsm/kg).

Management

There are two aspects to the management of hypernatraemia:

1. Stop any ongoing excessive loss of EFW.
2. Replace the EFW loss with hypotonic fluids (5% dextrose, oral water, half-normal saline) at an appropriate rate.

If the patient has significant volume depletion in addition to hypernatraemia (osmotic diuresis, diarrhoea), this should first be corrected

Table 1.4 Causes of diabetes insipidus

	Central	Nephrogenic
Congenital	Autosomal dominant (mutations in vasopressin precursor) Autosomal recessive (Wolfram syndrome)	X-linked (mutations in V2 receptor) Autosomal recessive (mutations in aquaporin 2)
Acquired	Tumours (pituitary, metastases) Postsurgery, head trauma Infiltration of the pituitary (sarcoid, histiocytosis) CNS infections Idiopathic (50%)	Chronic renal failure Renal interstitial disease (interstitial nephritis, obstructive uropathy, polycystic kidney disease, lithium therapy, sickle cell anaemia) Electrolyte disorders (hypokalaemia, hypercalcaemia) Drugs (lithium, amphotericin, foscarnet)

with normal saline. Great care must be taken with polyuric patients as any changes in urine osmolality or urine volume can rapidly change the serum sodium concentration, which needs frequent monitoring. The correction of hypernatraemia should not occur too rapidly as this may precipitate cerebral oedema and seizures. In general the hypernatraemia should be corrected over more than 48 h and no faster than 1–2 mmol/h.

Non-renal EFW loss

This is the commonest situation found in hospitalised patients as insensible losses can be large, especially if the patient is ventilated, febrile, etc. The key to successful management is the accurate estimation of all EFW losses (respiratory, sweat, gastrointestinal) and to match these losses with the appropriate intravenous fluids. This will prevent worsening of the hypernatraemia whilst additional EFW must then be given to correct the hypernatraemia. The water deficit can be calculated from the equation:

$$\text{Water deficit} = \frac{(\text{Serum[Na]} - 140)}{140} \times \text{Total body water}$$

This may be a useful guide to therapy. Typically half of the calculated water deficit may be replaced within the first 24 h.

Osmotic diuresis

Therapy should be directed at treating the underlying cause (e.g. insulin for hyperglycaemia) in order to reduce the excess EFW losses. There is often significant volume depletion, which should be corrected with normal saline. Half-normal saline is usually used as a source of EFW in hyperglycaemia to correct the hypernatraemia as 5% dextrose may exacerbate the raised blood sugar.

Central diabetes insipidus

This responds to ADH replacement therapy, which is usually administered as intranasal desmopressin acetate (10–20 µg once or twice per day). The patient should reduce oral water intake while receiving this therapy or hyponatraemia will develop.

Nephrogenic diabetes insipidus

The underlying cause should be treated e.g. hypercalcaemia or hypokalaemia and any contributing drugs such lithium discontinued if possible. Often, nephrogenic diabetes insipidus is due to chronic interstitial renal disease, which may not be reversible. In such circumstances the maintenance of a high oral water intake will maintain the serum sodium level in the normal range but at the expense of polyuria. Measures to decrease the polyuria include dietary changes (low sodium intake, protein restriction) and drugs that interfere with urine dilution such as thiazide diuretics.

Assessment of polyuria

Subjects with abnormal water balance and polyuria can maintain normal serum sodium concentrations by matching their EFW losses with adequate water intake. These patients present with polyuria rather than hypernatraemia. The polyuria, generally defined as more than 3 L urine per day, should be confirmed by measuring at least two 24-h urine collections. Laboratory testing should include estimation of plasma sodium, potassium, calcium and glucose levels, and plasma osmolality. Urine tests should include osmolality and urine electrolytes (sodium, potassium, chloride and urea) and testing for glycosuria. The polyuria should be considered to be due to a water diuresis or a solute diuresis, although both may be present in the same patient.

Water diuresis

In this setting, the polyuria is due to excess urine water loss (diabetes insipidus, psychogenic polydipsia). Therefore, the 24-h osmole excretion rate is normal ($\sim$10 mOsm/kg/day). It can be difficult to differentiate between diabetes insipidus and psychogenic polydipsia. A water deprivation test and measurement of plasma ADH levels may need to be performed.

Solute diuresis

In this setting, the polyuria is driven by excess solute excretion (glycosuria, high sodium intake (i.v. saline, high salt diet) or, more rarely, high urea excretion (patients who are catabolic, receiving high protein feeds or recovering from acute renal failure). Correcting the source of the excess solute will treat the cause of polyuria, and hypotonic fluids will correct the hypernatraemia.

CHAPTER 2

Disorders of potassium balance

The body in steady state is in potassium balance with potassium intake (normally 60–80 mmol/d) equal to potassium excretion (renal excretion 50–65 mmol/d and stool 10–15 mmol/d). The normal serum potassium concentration ranges from 3.5 to 5.0 mmol/L.

Learning point

Disturbances of plasma potassium (K) levels are commonly encountered in clinical practice. Both hyperkalaemia and hypokalaemia may be life-threatening medical emergencies.

Distribution

Some 98% of total body potassium is intracellular and this is maintained by the Na–K-ATPase pump (Fig. 2.1). Therefore, a significant shift in potassium to or from the intracellular fluid (ICF) can markedly affect the serum potassium concentration and exert profound effects on the resting membrane potential.

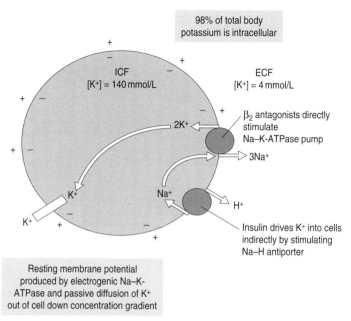

98% of total body
potassium is intracellular

ICF
$[K^+] = 140$ mmol/L

ECF
$[K^+] = 4$ mmol/L

$2K^+$

β_2 antagonists directly stimulate Na–K-ATPase pump

$3Na^+$

K^+

Na^+

H^+

K^+

Insulin drives K^+ into cells indirectly by stimulating Na–H antiporter

Resting membrane potential produced by electrogenic Na–K-ATPase and passive diffusion of K^+ out of cell down concentration gradient

Figure 2.1 Potassium distribution and resting membrane potential. Some 98% of potassium is intracellular. The resting membrane potential is produced by the electrogenic Na–K-ATPase and passive diffusion of K^+ out of the cell down the concentration gradient. ICF, intracellular fluid; ECF, extracellular fluid.

Example:

A 70-kg man contains 42L total body water, 14L extracellular fluid and 28L intracellular fluid.

Total ECF potassium $= 14 \times 4.0 = 56$ mmol
Total ICF potassium $= 28 \times 140 = 3920$ mmol

Potassium excretion

The kidney is primarily responsible for potassium regulation. In health, the kidney can lower renal excretion to 5–10 mmol per day or increase excretion to 450 mmol per day depending upon potassium intake.

Renal potassium excretion

Under normal circumstances, 180 L plasma are filtered per day, resulting in the entry of 720 mmol potassium into the lumen of the nephron. If the serum K concentration increases to 5.0 mmol/L, then an extra 180 mmol K will be filtered. The majority of the filtered K (around 500 mmol) is reabsorbed in the proximal tubule. The control of potassium secretion occurs primarily in the principal cells of the cortical collecting duct (CCD) (Fig. 2.2). Potassium secretion is dependent on the delivery of sodium and water to the CCD and on the action of the hormone aldosterone. Aldosterone increases sodium reabsorption from the lumen and promotes potassium secretion into the lumen, restoring electrical neutrality.

Gastrointestinal potassium excretion

Although gastrointestinal loss usually accounts for 10–15 mmol K excretion per day, this route can be increased in chronic renal failure, when it may account for up to 50% of potassium intake.

When should I check potassium level?

There are myriad potential reasons for requesting estimation of a serum potassium (K) level but the commonest and most important indications in clinical practice include the following.

Patients with cardiac disease

Both raised (hyperkalaemia) and subnormal (hypokalaemia) serum potassium levels may have significant effects upon cardiac conduction. It is therefore critically important to ensure that potassium levels are maintained in the normal range in patients with myocardial infarction, cardiac dysrhythmias or receiving digoxin therapy.

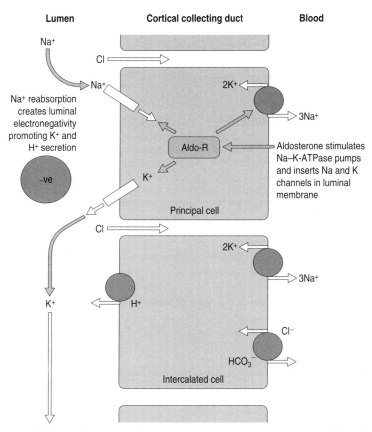

Figure 2.2 Renal excretion of potassium. Potassium secretion is controlled in the cortical collecting duct (CCD). Sodium reabsorption in this segment produces a negative voltage gradient, promoting K secretion under the actions of aldosterone. Aldo-R, aldosterone receptor.

Patients receiving drugs that may affect serum potassium level

Drugs such as loop diuretics may lower serum potassium levels, whereas drugs such as potassium-sparing diuretics, angiotensin converting enzyme (ACE) inhibitors, non-steroidal anti-inflammatory drugs (NSAIDs) may increase serum potassium levels.

Patients with diabetes mellitus

Patients who present to hospital with acute diabetic ketoacidosis often have normal or slightly raised potassium levels as the systemic acidosis promotes the exit of potassium from cells into the extracellular fluid. Treatment with insulin drives potassium back into the intracellular compartment and the serum potassium level may rapidly fall such that hypokalaemia is a real risk. These dehydrated patients typically receive large volumes of intravenous fluid and are markedly polyuric. They therefore require very close monitoring of serum potassium level (2–4-hourly) combined with judicious potassium supplementation. Patients with long-standing diabetes mellitus may also develop a type IV renal tubular acidosis, which may lead to troublesome hyperkalaemia. This often results in an intolerance to ACE inhibitors and to renal replacement therapy being commenced slightly earlier in diabetic patients than in patients with other causes of renal failure.

Patients with major fluid and electrolyte fluxes

This may be seen in patients receiving large volume of intravenous fluids, e.g. postsurgical patients with major fluid losses from drains and wounds as well as patients receiving total parenteral nutrition. In addition, severe diarrhoea may cause significant fluid and electrolyte disturbance with hypokalaemia.

Patients with renal impairment

Patients with renal functional impairment have a reduced capacity to excrete potassium and are therefore more prone to hyperkalaemia. A low threshold for checking serum potassium is recommended in such patients, particularly if a potential cause for hyperkalaemia is present.

Patients with weakness of unknown aetiology

Potassium plays an important role in neuromuscular physiology, and paralysis and ventilatory respiratory failure may ensue from severe hypokalaemia.

What do I do with the result?

Usually, the potassium level does not require overt action, although trends should be sought, i.e. if the potassium level is 'drifting up' then look for a cause and deal with it. Is the patient receiving potassium supplements? Is the patient's renal function normal? However, anything other than prompt action when potassium levels are below 3 mmol/L or greater than 6 mmol/L is perilous. The management of these important scenarios is outlined later in this chapter.

Hypokalaemia (<3.5 mmol/L)

Hypokalaemia may result from depletion of total body potassium secondary to excessive renal or gastrointestinal losses, but may also result from a shift of potassium into cells.

Symptoms and signs

> The primary symptoms of hypokalaemia are muscle weakness and paraesthesia. The primary risks are cardiac arrhythmias and ventilatory failure.

Hypokalaemia results in hyperpolarisation of the cell membrane, which impairs the ability of the cell to generate action potentials in excitable tissues such as muscles and nerves. Mild hypokalaemia (3–3.5 mmol/L) is often asymptomatic. Moderate hypokalaemia (2.5–3.0 mmol/L) may result in muscle weakness, fatigue and paraesthesia as well as ileus and constipation, because the smooth muscle of the gastrointestinal tract may be affected. In rare instances, severe hypokalaemia may precipitate rhabdomyolysis. Hypokalaemia may also interfere with the ability of the kidney to concentrate the urine, thereby resulting in nephrogenic diabetes insipidus with polyuria and polydipsia.

In patients with cardiac disease, hypokalaemia is associated with a greatly increased risk of ventricular arrhythmias. Although ECG changes (flattened T waves, inverted T waves, U waves) are typically present when the serum potassium level is less than 3.0 mmol/L, these changes do not correlate well with the risk of ventricular arrhythmias (Fig. 2.3). Severe hypokalaemia (<2.5 mmol/L) can lead to weakness of respiratory muscles and ventilatory failure.

Differential diagnosis

Hypokalaemia may be considered to be due to insufficient potassium intake, a shift of potassium from the extracellular fluid to the intracellular compartment or excessive potassium excretion from the gut or kidneys.

Artefactual

This may occur if the blood was drawn from near the site of an intravenous infusion of fluid that does not contain potassium. In cases of doubt, take another sample to confirm or refute the diagnosis.

Low potassium intake

This may be due to insufficient potassium in the diet or intravenous fluids (e.g. postsurgery). It should be noted that, as the fall in potassium intake induces increased renal conservation of potassium, a low potassium intake alone does not cause hypokalaemia.

Shift of potassium into the intracellular compartment

Factors stimulating a shift of potassium into cells include insulin, β_2 agonists such as salbutamol, catecholamines or an alkalosis. Hypokalaemia may therefore occur in patients receiving treatment for diabetes mellitus or asthma. It should also be noted that concurrent hypophosphataemia is suggestive of an intracellular shift of potassium.

Gastrointestinal losses

Gastrointestinal losses such as vomiting, nasogastric aspiration or diarrhoea are a common cause of hypokalaemia. Interestingly, the potassium concentration of gastric juice is only 10 mmol/L, but the vomiting is often associated with extracellular volume contraction. This stimulates aldosterone release and, combined with the increased delivery of sodium bicarbonate to the distal nephron, results in renal potassium wasting. The potassium concentration in diarrhoea is often 30–35 mmol/L, and the hypokalaemia that may result is associated with a non-anion gap metabolic acidosis. Other causes of gastrointestinal potassium loss include villous adenomas, fistulae, laxative abuse and ureterosigmoidostomy.

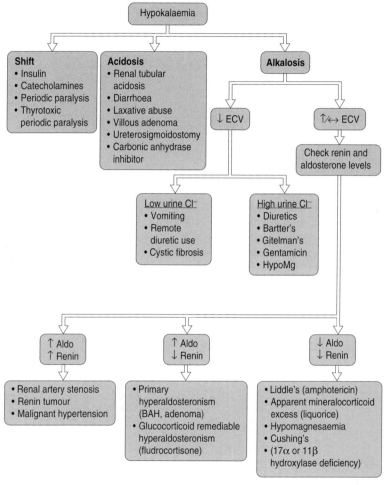

Figure 2.3 Differential diagnosis of hypokalaemia. Aldo, aldosterone; BAH, bilateral adrenal hyperplasia; ECV, extracellular fluid volume; hypoMg, hypomagnesaemia.

Renal losses

Diuretics are the most common cause of hypokalaemia. They inhibit sodium reabsorption resulting in extracellular volume contraction with stimulation of aldosterone release, and increase the delivery of sodium and chloride to the CCD. Bartter's and Gitelman's syndromes are rare genetic conditions in which mutations in genes encoding sodium transporters in the loop of Henle and distal tubule respectively simulate chronic diuretic use.

Drugs associated with hypokalaemia:

Diuretics, gentamicin, amphotericin, carbenoxolone, laxatives, acetazolamide, fludrocortisone

---

Hyperaldosteronism secondary to a decreased extracellular volume promotes renal potassium loss. In primary hyperaldosteronism there is autonomous aldosterone production from an adrenal adenoma or bilateral adrenal hyperplasia resulting in expansion of extracellular volume and an increased delivery of sodium and chloride to the CCD. The sodium and water retention results in hypertension with a characteristic hypokalaemic metabolic alkalosis. Other causes of excess mineralocorticoid activity include Cushing's syndrome and exogenous corticosteroids or fludrocortisone.

Although renal diseases that result in renal failure are typically associated with hyperkalaemia due to a decreased glomerular filtration rate, some renal disorders are associated with hypokalaemia. For example, renal tubular acidosis (RTA) results in increased urinary potassium loss as well as causing a chronic systemic acidosis. The increased urinary potassium loss results from distal potassium secretion secondary to either increased sodium delivery to the distal tubule (proximal RTA) or defective distal hydrogen ion excretion (distal RTA).

Special situations

Heart disease

In patients with cardiac disease, e.g. postmyocardial infarction and cardiac failure (particularly if taking digoxin), hypokalaemia may induce ventricular arrhythmias and the serum potassium level should be maintained at the high end of normal.

Liver failure

Hypokalaemia results in increased production of ammonia and can exacerbate hepatic encephalopathy.

Management

Assessment

The presence of paralysis or arrhythmias indicates an emergency situation. Assess the cardiovascular status (pulse rate, rhythm, lying and standing blood pressure, jugular venous pressure, presence of oedema) and look for evidence of arrhythmias (check ECG) and hypo/hypervolaemia. Is the patient diabetic or asthmatic? Carefully scrutinise the fluid balance charts – is the patient oliguric and in renal failure? Examine the drug chart for drugs that can affect potassium levels, e.g. insulin, diuretics, steroids, gentamicin. Does the patient have an abnormal venous bicarbonate level indicating a metabolic acidosis or alkalosis? Consider the degree of potassium deficit and ongoing potassium losses from gastrointestinal tract or kidneys. Check the serum magnesium level in complicated patients or in those with severe hypokalaemia, as hypokalaemia will not respond to replacement therapy if the patient is hypomagnesaemic.

Emergency treatment

- If hypokalaemia is severe (<2.5 mmol/L) it may be associated with muscle weakness leading to ventilatory failure or cardiac arrhythmias. Intravenous replacement is appropriate in this setting.
- Potassium chloride should be diluted in normal saline to a concentration of ≤40–60 mmol/L. Note that dextrose solutions may stimulate insulin and shift potassium into cells and should not be used. Rarely 10–20 mmol potassium chloride (KCl) may be infused in 100 mL saline over 30 min in extreme situations. **Never give ampoules of KCl directly without diluting.** Potassium-containing intravenous solutions can be very irritant to peripheral veins and it may be preferable to give these through a central line.
- The initial rate of potassium replacement may be as high as 20–40 mmol/h, but this should be done only with continuous ECG monitoring. The replacement rate should be reduced to

10 mmol/h when the patient is out of immediate danger. The serum potassium must be checked regularly (initially at least hourly) during emergency treatment.

Non-urgent treatment

- Any underlying conditions such as renal failure should be treated and causative drugs discontinued.
- Oral potassium replacement is the safest route for potassium replacement in most situations, although potassium supplements may cause gastrointestinal upset. Typical replacement in the short term may be 60–120 mmol potassium chloride per day in three or four divided doses. Attention should be paid to ongoing potassium losses, and treatment should be guided by serum potassium measurements.

Hyperkalaemia

Hyperkalaemia is often asymptomatic, but the primary risk is of cardiac arrhythmias and sudden death.

Symptoms and signs

Hyperkalaemia reduces the polarisation of the cell membrane so that it falls closer to the threshold for depolarisation, thereby making cells more excitable. Clinical symptoms are uncommon, although some patients may experience paraesthesia, cramps, severe muscle weakness or even paralysis.

The main danger is cardiac arrhythmia, particularly bradyarrhythmias or sudden death. The risk is related to the degree of hyperkalaemia (>6.0 mmol/L), the rate of rise of the serum potassium level and the degree of acidosis or hypoxia. ECG changes including tall peaked T waves are typically present, but more worrisome changes include bradycardia, prolongation of the PR interval, loss of P waves, broadening of the QRS complex and the development of a 'sine wave' pattern (Fig. 2.4).

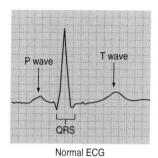

Normal ECG

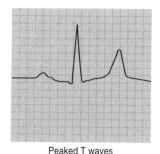

Peaked T waves

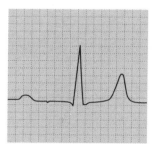

Prolonged PR interval

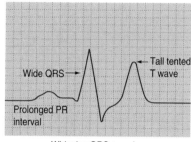

Widening QRS complex

Figure 2.4 ECG changes of hyperkalaemia.

Special situations

Diabetic ketoacidosis

Hyperkalaemia may occur at presentation due to a shift of potassium out of cells (due to insulin lack and hyperglycaemia). However, total body potassium is depleted due to prior urinary loss of K (osmotic diuresis and loss with keto-anions) and serum potassium levels can fall precipitously when insulin and IV fluids are commenced.

Differential diagnosis (Fig. 2.5)

The most common causes of hyperkalaemia are
- Acute or chronic renal impairment with consequent reduced potassium excretion
- Drug related
- Acute shifts of potassium out of cells into the extracellular fluid.

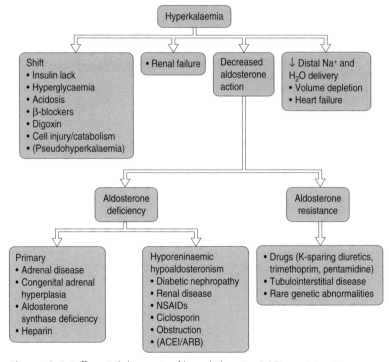

Figure 2.5 Differential diagnosis of hyperkalaemia. ACEI, angiotensin-converting enzyme inhibitors; ARB, angiotensin II receptor blockers; NSAIDs, non-steroidal anti-inflammatory drugs.

Artefactual and pseudohyperkalaemia

This may occur if the venesection was traumatic or there was a long delay (>3 h) between venesection and separation of the plasma, as potassium may leak slowly from cells. Consider pseudohyperkalaemia in situations where there is a marked leukocytosis (>11 × 10^6/mL) or thrombocytosis (>400 × 10^6/mL). In this case the serum K concentration will be raised but the plasma K level will be normal.

High potassium intake

Increased potassium intake *per se* is not a cause of hyperkalaemia as the kidneys can excrete a large potassium load. A high potassium intake, however, may be a significant contributing factor especially in patients with impaired renal function. High intake may be dietary (fruits, certain vegetables) or iatrogenic (secondary to excessive K replacement).

Shift of potassium from the intracellular compartment

Factors promoting a shift of potassium out of cells include hyperglycaemia, a lack of insulin, β_2 antagonists and acidosis. Note that the combination of hyperphosphataemia and hyperkalaemia is found in conditions associated with cell damage such as rhabdomyolysis, severe burns, tumour lysis syndrome or following severe blood transfusion reactions.

Reduced renal potassium excretion

This is most commonly due to renal failure or to drugs that interfere with potassium excretion.

Drugs associated with hyperkalaemia

ACE inhibitors, angiotensin II receptor blockers, potassium-sparing diuretics, NSAIDs, digoxin, β_2 antagonists, ciclosporin.

Renal potassium excretion requires an adequate glomerular filtration rate, delivery of sodium to the distal nephron and the action of aldosterone (see Fig. 2.2).

- A decreased glomerular filtration rate is found in acute and chronic renal failure.

- Reduced sodium delivery to the distal nephron may be seen with severe volume depletion or heart failure – the urine sodium concentration is low (<20 mmol/L).
- Impaired aldosterone action may be due to adrenal disease (e.g. Addison's disease, hyporeninaemic hypoaldosteronism) or aldosterone resistance (e.g. potassium-sparing diuretics, tubulointerstitial disease, obstructive nephropathy). It should be noted that diabetic patients with diabetic nephropathy may develop hyporeninaemic hypoaldosteronism and troublesome hyperkalaemia at an earlier stage than non-diabetic patients with chronic renal impairment, often necessitating the institution of renal replacement therapy at an earlier stage.

Management

Assessment

If the serum potassium is >6.5 mmol/L then emergency treatment is merited. Check the ECG trace for signs of cardiac instability and proceed to emergency treatment if ECG changes are present. Assess the patient's cardiovascular status (pulse rate and rhythm, lying and sitting/standing blood pressure, jugular venous pressure, presence of oedema) for evidence of arrhythmias and hypo/hypervolaemia. Is the patient diabetic? What is the blood glucose level? Is the patient hypoxic or acidotic? Check the urine output and the drug chart carefully for drugs that may be implicated in raising the potassium level.

Emergency treatment (Table 2.1)

If ECG reveals changes of hyperkalaemia, continue ECG monitoring and obtain intravenous access.

1. Give intravenous calcium gluconate (10%, 10 mL administered over 5 min) to antagonise the effects of hyperkalaemia on the heart and stabilise the myocardium. This drug is short acting and may need to be repeated.
2. Shift potassium into cells by giving insulin and dextrose (6 units fast-acting insulin and 50 mL 50% dextrose) over 10 min. Commence an insulin and dextrose infusion (6 units fast-acting insulin, 50 mL 50% dextrose in 500 mL 5% dextrose) with monitoring of blood glucose levels. If the patient is acidotic and not in pulmonary oedema, consider giving sodium bicarbonate (500 mL 1.4% $NaHCO_3$

Table 2.1 Emergency therapy of hyperkalaemia

Therapy	Dose	Mechanism of action	Onset	Duration of action	Risks
Calcium gluconate	10 mL of 10%	Stabilises myocardium	1 min	10–20 min	Vein irritation
Insulin and dextrose	50 mL 50% + 6 units insulin	Shifts K^+ into cells	20–30 min	2 h	Hypoglycaemia
Sodium bicarbonate	500 mL of 1.4%	Shifts K^+ into cells	2–4 h	Up to 24 h	Volume overload
Salbutamol	20 mg in 4 mL saline nebulised	Shifts K^+ into cells	15–30 min	2 h	Tachycardia
Calcium resonium	15 g t.i.d. (with 30 mL lactulose)	Binds K^+ in bowel	2–4 h	Removes K^+	Intestinal obstruction
Haemodialysis	–	Removes K^+	30 min	Removes K^+	

over 1–2 h). Note that 8.4% $NaHCO_3$ is hypertonic and should not be given peripherally. If central venous access is available, consider giving aliquots of 25–50 mL 8.4% $NaHCO_3$ but monitor carefully for volume overload. β_2 agonists such as salbutamol will also shift potassium into cells, but may exacerbate cardiac instability and are usually used in children.

3. Increase potassium elimination by giving cation exchange resin (15 g calcium resonium with 30 mL lactulose three times per day). This is a slow-acting treatment and not appropriate in an emergency setting.

4. Dialysis may be required in patients with renal failure and refractory hyperkalaemia.

Non-urgent treatment

Any underlying causes should be treated, offending drugs discontinued and a low potassium diet considered. Long-term therapy with cation exchange resins should be avoided as there is a risk of forming concretions in the bowel. Increased renal potassium elimination may be achieved by volume expansion with normal saline and judicious use of loop diuretics to improve the distal delivery of sodium and water. Fludrocortisone may be useful in the setting of hypoaldosteronism.

CHAPTER 3

Assessment of renal function and urinary protein excretion

Introduction

The assessment of renal function is important in both inpatient and outpatient settings. Renal function is generally assessed by measuring the serum creatinine and urea levels, or calculating the glomerular filtration rate (GFR) (or creatinine clearance). Acute renal failure occurs when renal function deteriorates over a short period of time (days to weeks) and is common in patients in intensive care units as a complication of conditions such as septic shock, pancreatitis, etc. Chronic renal failure is irreversible renal impairment that commonly occurs in patients with medical conditions such as diabetes, ischaemic heart disease and long-standing hypertension, and must be taken into account in their clinical management. It is important to note that, in conditions that are limited to the kidneys, the only clinical evidence of disease may be the presence of haematuria, proteinuria and/or renal impairment. Therefore the pertinent investigations covered in this chapter will include:

- Measurement of serum creatinine and urea levels, and creatinine clearance
- Dipstick urinalysis for blood and protein
- Urinary protein excretion and estimation.

Learning point

Many seriously ill, hospitalised patients develop a degree of renal failure and the early detection of impaired renal function facilitates the initiation of relevant clinical investigations, appropriate management of fluid and drug therapy, and may prevent a requirement for dialysis.

The incidence of renal failure is increasing inexorably, with the elderly population being particularly affected. These individuals exhibit a range of conditions including renovascular disease and prostatic obstruction, as well as diabetic nephropathy or acute glomerulonephritis.

It is pertinent to consider the normal function of the kidneys as this provides insights into what may become deranged in disease. In health the kidneys are responsible for maintaining salt and water, potassium, phosphate and acid–base homeostasis as well as producing the hormones 1,25-dihydroxycholecalciferol (active vitamin D) and erythropoietin, which stimulates the production of erythrocytes. It is therefore predictable that patients with failing kidneys may exhibit salt and water retention (hypertension, oedema), hyperkalaemia, hyperphosphataemia, a metabolic acidosis (low venous bicarbonate), a raised parathyroid hormone level, hypocalcaemia and anaemia, as well as increased levels of urea and creatinine.

Assessment of renal function

Serum creatinine

Creatinine is a nitrogenous waste product produced from creatine in muscle and is excreted by the kidneys. The majority of creatinine is excreted by glomerular filtration, but a small portion (~10%) is secreted into the proximal tubular lumen. The normal serum concentration of creatinine varies considerably between individuals (60–120 µmol/L), depending on muscle mass, and can be used to estimate renal function.

Serum creatinine levels may be increased in

- Impaired renal function (renal failure). This is the most common cause.
- Individuals with a large muscle mass, e.g. body builders
- Individuals taking certain drugs, such as trimethoprim or cimetidine, as these can interfere with the renal tubular handling of creatinine.

The serum creatinine may be low in

- Patients with a low muscle mass (malnourished, wasting and debilitating diseases, or frail elderly individuals)
- Pregnant women (as a result of the increased GFR).

It must be emphasised that the serum creatinine level *per se* (normal range 60–120 µmol/L) is not an accurate measure of renal function, as the serum creatinine level does not become raised until more than 50% of renal function has been lost. It is therefore an insensitive marker of the early stages of renal impairment as large changes in

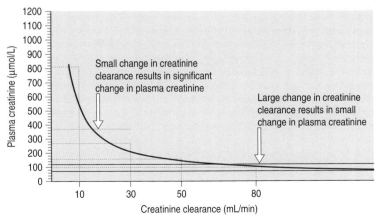

Figure 3.1 Relationship between plasma creatinine and creatinine clearance.

GFR result in small changes in serum creatinine concentration (Fig. 3.1). The serum creatinine level may, however, be used to track the progression of established acute or chronic renal failure. In particular, a graphical plot of 1/plasma creatinine against time (a reciprocal creatinine plot) approximates to a straight line and the line may be extrapolated to intersect the x-axis (time) and provide an estimate of when the patient will reach end-stage renal disease if the rate of deterioration in renal function remains constant (Fig. 3.2). The slope of the reciprocal creatinine plot is very important: if the slope increases, this indicates that the rate of loss of renal function has accelerated and the patient will require dialysis earlier. Conversely, if the slope diminishes then this indicates a diminution in the rate of progression of renal failure. Figure 3.2 depicts the reciprocal creatinine plot of a patient with hypertensive renal disease who has progressive renal impairment. An increased rate of deterioration was secondary to a period of uncontrolled severe hypertension, although eventually the hypertension was controlled by a change in treatment. Comparison of the extrapolated lines demonstrates that the regaining of blood pressure control will have a major impact upon the eventual timing of the requirement for dialysis.

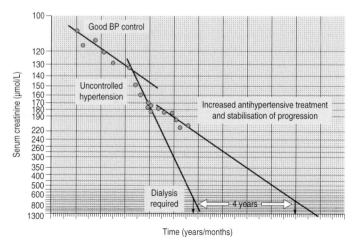

Figure 3.2 The reciprocal creatinine plot.

Serum urea

Serum urea is of much less value than the serum creatinine level in the assessment of renal function as the urea level is determined by many variables other than renal function. Urea is a product of protein metabolism and is generated in the liver following the deamination of amino acids. Urea is excreted by the kidneys, undergoing glomerular filtration, but approximately 50% is then reabsorbed. The normal urea concentration is 2.5–6.6 mmol/L, but is highly dependent on protein intake and volume status.

The serum urea concentration may be raised in

- Impaired renal function (renal failure)
- Volume depletion (increases renal reabsorption of urea)
- High protein diet
- Upper gastrointestinal bleed (protein load and hypovolaemia)
- Catabolic states (sepsis, steroid therapy).

The serum urea concentration may be decreased in

- Reduced protein intake (starvation, anorexia)
- Malabsorption
- Liver disease (unable to generate urea).

Of note, a disproportionate rise in the level of urea or creatinine in acute renal failure may give a clue to the underlying disorder. Serum creatinine levels may be increased when urea levels are relatively normal owing to decreased protein intake. Acute muscle injury (rhabdomyolysis) may cause acute renal failure (see Chapter 9), and in this setting the serum creatinine concentration may be disporportionately raised (muscle injury). By contrast, a disproportionate increase in the serum urea level may suggest volume depletion (secondary to increased urea reabsorption).

Glomerular filtration rate and creatinine clearance

Approximately 180 L of plasma water are filtered per day as blood passes through the microvascular networks of the two to three million glomeruli that are present in normal kidneys. This glomerular filtration rate (GFR) depends upon the number of functioning glomeruli, the intraglomerular hydrostatic pressure, and the nature and surface area of glomerular filtration surface. Disease may affect any or all of these variables.

The normal GFR is approximately 100 mL per min per 1.73 m² body surface area, although the normal range is wide and varies with age (Table 3.1). The GFR may be measured by various clearance techniques. The clearance of any substance can be calculated by the equation:

$$C = (U \times V)/P$$

where U is the urine concentration of the substance, V is the urine flow rate and P is the plasma concentration. When the substance is freely filtered at the glomerulus and is neither reabsorbed nor secreted by the tubules, the clearance of that substance is equal to the GFR. Inulin, iohexol, ^{51}Cr-EDTA or ^{99}Tc-DTPA may be used accurately to measure GFR by this methodology, but this requires the intravenous administration of the chosen filtration marker and is not performed routinely.

The clearance of creatinine over a 24-h period may be calculated using a 24-h urine collection (urine volume and creatinine concentration) and a serum creatinine measurement. The 24-h creatinine clearance is used in clinical practice to give a useful, albeit approximate, measure of the GFR. Creatinine is freely filtered at the glomerulus but is also secreted by the tubules to a limited extent (~10%), and thus the creatinine clearance overestimates the GFR, particularly in the setting of advanced renal impairment where secretion of creatinine constitutes a larger proportion of creatinine excretion. Another factor that limits the exactness of the creatinine clearance is the potential inaccuracy of any timed urine collection, which can vary by 20–30%.

Table 3.1 Normal GFR at different ages

Age (years)	GFR (mL per min per 1.73 m²)
20–30	116
30–40	107
40–50	99
50–60	93
60–70	85
70+	75

Table 3.2 Stages of chronic kidney disease

Stage	GFR (mL/min)	Level of renal function	Comments
1	>90	Normal renal function	Requires the presence of proteinuria, microscopic haematuria or abnormal renal structure, e.g. genetic disease or evidence of renal injury or scarring
2	60–89	Mild renal impairment	Requires the presence of proteinuria, microscopic haematuria or abnormal renal structure, e.g. genetic disease or evidence of renal injury or scarring
3	30–59	Moderate renal impairment	
4	15–29	Severe renal impairment	Consider active planning for end-stage renal disease
5	<15	Approaching or at end-stage renal failure	Consider renal replacement therapy (haemodialysis or peritoneal dialysis), renal transplantation or conservative management

Stages of chronic kidney disease

The GFR is used to categorise the stage of chronic kidney disease (CKD), as indicated in Table 3.2. Note that the presence of proteinuria, haematuria, genetic renal disease (e.g. polycystic renal disease) or evidence of renal injury on a renal biopsy results in individuals being classified as having stage 1 CKD even if the GFR is completely normal.

Equations to estimate glomerular filtration rate

As indicated above, the creatinine clearance is commonly measured by using a 24-h urine collection, but this does introduce the potential for error in terms of the completeness of the collection. An alternative and more convenient method is to employ various formulae devised to calculate the creatinine clearance using parameters such as serum creatinine level, sex, age and weight of the patient. An example is the Cockcroft and Gault formula:

$$GFR = \frac{K \times (140 - Age) \times Bodyweight}{Serum\ creatinine\ (\mu mol/L)}$$

where K is a constant that varies with sex: 1.23 for males and 1.04 for females. The constant K is used as females have a relatively lower muscle mass. The Cockcroft and Gault formula overestimates the GFR if the patient is obese.

An alternative formula for calculating GFR from the serum creatinine is the Modification of Diet in Renal Disease (MDRD) formula, which does not use the patient's weight for the calculation of GFR. The formula uses the serum levels of urea, creatinine and albumin together with age and various correction coefficients for sex and race. There are limitations to the use of the MDRD formula and it has not been validated in elderly patients, pregnant women, children or patients with marked hypoalbuminaemia. Despite these caveats, it is of use in adult medicine and some laboratories are including the value for the 'estimated GFR' (eGFR) derived from the MDRD formula on clinical chemistry reports. An MDRD GFR calculator can be accessed online at http://www.kidney.org/professionals/KDOQI/gfr_calculator.cfm.

The inaccuracy of using the serum creatinine level in isolation as an indicator of renal function is demonstrated by calculating the estimated creatinine clearance using such equations. Using the Cockcroft and Gault formula, the estimated GFR of a 55-year-old man weighing 100 kg with a serum creatinine level of 230 μmol/L is 46 mL/min (stage 3 CKD). In contrast, a 55-year-old woman weighing 44 kg with a serum creatinine level of 230 μmol/L has an estimated GFR of 16 mL/min (stage 4 CKD, and very near to stage 5). This very marked difference in renal function would have a major impact on patient management and results from the fact that the serum creatinine level is related to muscle mass. There are numerous examples of malnourished small older women with significant renal impairment but a serum creatinine level that is not far outside the 'normal range'.

Other examples using the MDRD formula are shown in Table 3.3. Of note, although renal function does deteriorate slightly with age, the serum creatinine concentration of elderly individuals should still be in the normal range. Thus, a raised serum creatinine level in an elderly individual is abnormal and merits further investigation.

Learning point

The serum creatinine concentration is of limited value on its own and must be considered in conjunction with the age and muscle mass of the patient. It may be used:

- to generate an estimated GFR using various formulae
- to track the individual progress of a patient over time using a reciprocal creatinine plot.

Table 3.3 Examples of GFR estimated from serum creatinine

Age (years)	Sex	Race	Serum creatinine (mol/L)	eGFR[a] (mL per min per 1.73 m^2)
25	M	Black	140	69
25	M	Caucasian	140	57
25	F	Caucasian	140	42
60	M	Caucasian	140	48
60	F	Black	140	43
60	F	Caucasian	140	35

[a]Glomerular filtration rate estimated by the Modification of Diet in Renal Disease (MDRD) Study equation.

Regulation of renal blood flow and the glomerular filtration rate

Renal autoregulation acts to maintain renal blood flow at a constant level despite fluctuations in the mean systemic arterial pressure. For example, the glomerulus is protected from the effects of systemic blood pressure due to reflex vasoconstriction of the afferent arteriole supplying the glomerulus. Afferent arteriolar vasoconstriction is also induced if there is increased delivery of sodium chloride to the macula densa at the end of the loop of Henle (as would happen as a result of an increase in systemic blood pressure, renal blood flow or GFR). There are also mechanisms to maintain the GFR in the face of diminished renal perfusion as may occur in hypovolaemic patients. Reduced renal perfusion results in prostaglandin-mediated dilatation of the afferent arteriole and angiotensin II-mediated vasoconstriction of the efferent arteriole exiting the glomerulus. This maintains intraglomerular hydrostatic filtration pressure and preserves the GFR (Fig. 3.3). Despite these protective mechanisms, the GFR will eventually fall in conditions associated with a prolonged or severe reduction in renal perfusion.

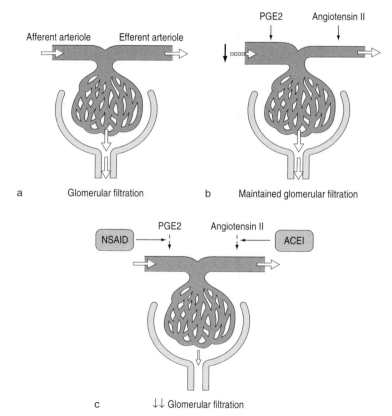

Figure 3.3 Glomerular filtration during (a) normal renal perfusion and (b) reduced renal perfusion. GFR is maintained by prostaglandin (PG)-mediated dilatation of the afferent arteriole, and angiotensin II-mediated vasoconstriction of the efferent arteriole. (c) Reduced filtration during reduced renal perfusion due to NSAID or ACE inhibitor (ACEI) treatment antagonising autoregulation.

An important clinical point is that many patients are treated with angiotensin-converting enzyme (ACE) inhibitors and non-steroidal anti-inflammatory drugs (NSAIDs), both of which are potentially dangerous in the setting of reduced renal perfusion. ACE inhibitor-mediated inhibition of efferent arteriolar vasoconstriction lowers the intraglomerular pressure and reduces nephron hyperfiltration. This may be beneficial in CKD as the decreased glomerular pressure will reduce proteinuria, which is a well documented risk factor for progression of renal disease. However, in the context of reduced renal perfusion (e.g. renal artery stenosis, hypovolaemia, severe heart failure), the reduction in the capacity of the kidney to maintain the GFR puts patients at an increased risk of developing acute renal failure. NSAIDs may also lead to acute renal failure in these settings by inhibiting the autoregulatory dilatation of the afferent arteriole by prostaglandins.

Learning point

Treatment with ACE inhibitors or NSAIDs reduces the capacity of the kidney to maintain the GFR during episodes of renal hypoperfusion, putting the patient at risk of acute renal failure.

Assessment of proteinuria

Both protein size and charge dictate whether proteins are filtered at the glomerulus under normal circumstances, with anionic proteins being filtered to a lesser extent than cationic proteins. Low molecular weight proteins are filtered in normal circumstances but are actively reabsorbed by proximal renal tubular cells. Thus, although 4–5 g protein is filtered per day, the normal urinary protein excretion is less than 300 mg per 24 h. Glomerular diseases damage the glomerular filtration barrier resulting in large amounts of urinary protein (predominantly albumin) excretion. By contrast, tubular injury impairs the reabsorption of low molecular weight proteins.

Classification of proteinuria

Microalbuminuria

This comprises an increased level of urinary albumin excretion that is insufficient to be positive on a urinary dipstick (a positive urinary dipstick analysis for protein is called 'macroalbuminuria'). Microalbuminuria is defined as the excretion of 30–300 mg albumin per 24 h that has been confirmed on at least two occasions over a 3-month period (Table 3.4). Microalbuminuria may be determined by analysing:

- A 24-h urine collection: an albumin excretion of 30–300 mg/day represents microalbuminuria.
- A timed urine collection (e.g. overnight): an albumin excretion rate of 20–200 μg/min represents microalbuminuria.
- A spot urine sample (e.g. early morning urine), when the level of albumin is expressed with reference to the amount of creatinine in order to control for variation in urine concentration. An 'albumin to creatinine ratio' (or ACR) of 30–300 mg/g creatinine (3–30 mg/mmol creatinine) represents microalbuminuria. Normal ACR values vary with sex, and this needs to be taken into account: normal ACR is <2.5 mg/mmol creatinine in males and <3.5 mg/mmol creatinine in females.

Patients with type 1 or 2 diabetes and microalbuminuria are at high risk of developing overt diabetic nephropathy and such patients merit aggressive blood pressure control with ACE inhibitors as well as tight glycaemic control and correction of dyslipidaemia. Microalbuminuria may also be found in patients with hypertension and cardiovascular disease, and is an independent risk factor for cardiovascular mortality.

Table 3.4 Urinary albumin excretion

	Normal	Microalbuminuria	Macroalbuminuria
Albumin excretion rate using a 24-h urine collection	<30 mg/day	30–300 mg/day	>300 mg/day
Albumin excretion rate using a timed urine collection	<20 μg/min	20–200 μg/min	>200 μg/min
Albumin creatinine ratio using a spot urine sample	<30 mg/g creatinine or <3 mg/mmol creatinine	30–300 mg/g creatinine or 3–30 mg/mmol creatinine	>300 mg/g creatinine or >30 mg/mmol creatinine

Benign proteinuria

This is typically transient and secondary to physical activity or fever. Some patients exhibit orthostatic proteinuria that is dependent upon posture (see below).

Glomerular proteinuria

This is secondary to abnormal permeability of the glomerular filtration barrier. It may be due to structural damage, e.g. immune complex deposition in membranous nephropathy, or alteration of the cationic charge of the glomerular basement membrane, as this facilitates glomerular filtration of albumin, e.g. minimal change disease. Severe glomerular proteinuria may cause the nephrotic syndrome – a triad of heavy proteinuria (>3.5 g/day), hypoalbuminaemia and peripheral oedema.

Tubular proteinuria

This is secondary to reduced reabsorption of low molecular proteins such as β_2-microglobulin. Tubular proteinuria is found in conditions such as renal tubular acidosis, interstitial nephritis and acute tubular necrosis, and is usually less than 2 g/day. Tubular proteinuria never causes the nephrotic syndrome.

Overflow proteinuria

This is secondary to raised serum levels of proteins, such that the filtered load simply exceeds the capacity of the tubules to reabsorb them. For example, patients with myeloma may exhibit high circulating levels of light chains that are secreted by the clonal population of B cells and this gives rise to light chains in the urine (Bence Jones protein). Similarly, myoglobin or amylase may be evident in the urine of patients with rhabdomyolysis or pancreatitis respectively.

When should I consider performing dipstick urinalysis?

Ideally, all patients should have the urine checked for the presence of microscopic haematuria and protein. It is important to note that renal inflammation is typically 'silent' in most renal pathologies, including the 'renal limited' forms of diseases such as vasculitis. In these circumstances, the only sign of ongoing severe renal disease may be dipstick haematuria and proteinuria. Dipstick urinalysis detects mainly urinary albumin as it is less sensitive to immunoglobulins and other urinary proteins. The dipstick results are graded from negative to 4+ and the values approximate to the urinary protein concentration as follows: <10 mg/dL, negative; 10–20 mg/dL, trace; ~30 mg/dL, 1+; ~100 mg/dL, 2+; ~300 mg/dL, 3+; ~1000 mg/dL, 4+. Dipstick urinalysis should be performed in:

- Patients with diabetes mellitus as they are at risk of developing diabetic nephropathy.
- Patients with peripheral oedema or hypoalbuminaemia as they may have the nephrotic syndrome.
- Patients with known renal disease under follow-up as it may be a useful indicator of disease progression, remission or relapse, e.g. patients with minimal change disease.
- Patients with renal impairment as it can inform the differential diagnosis. For example, a middle-aged patient with renal impairment but no haematuria or proteinuria would be extremely unlikely to have active glomerulonephritis, and conditions such as renovascular disease or interstitial renal disease would need to be considered.
- Patients with immunological conditions such as systemic lupus erythematosus (SLE) as the onset of haematuria or proteinuria may be the first sign of renal involvement. Indeed, such patients may have significant renal disease that requires aggressive treatment despite having a completely normal plasma creatinine level.

Note that Bence Jones protein is not detected by urine dipstick analysis and requires specific immunoelectrophoresis of the urine. In addition, patients with a negative finding on dipstick urinalysis may still merit testing for microalbuminuria, for example patients with type 1 diabetes (after 5 years of disease), patients with newly diagnosed type 2 diabetes, or patients with cardiovascular disease or hypertension.

What do I do with the result?

Quantify the amount of proteinuria

All patients with persistent proteinuria on dipstick urinalysis require accurate quantification of protein excretion. This can be performed using a 24-h urine collection, but such collections may be inaccurate as patients may not collect all of the urine passed! Measurement of the urinary albumin/creatinine ratio on a spot urine sample is a useful and convenient method of determining the level of protein excretion. The correction for urine creatinine attempts to take into account the

Table 3.5 Conversion of protein/creatinine ratio to 24-h urinary protein excretion

Protein excretion (g/24 h)	Protein/creatinine ratio (mg/mmol creatinine)
<0.3	<30
1	100
3.5 (nephrotic range proteinuria)	350
10	1000

variation in urine concentration that occurs during the day. Table 3.5 shows the approximate conversions for a 70-kg man, although it should be noted that the muscle mass of the patient and the rate of creatinine production, and hence of excretion, will affect the values obtained. Therefore, individuals with a higher creatinine production will have a lower protein/creatinine ratio for a particular level of proteinuria. Ideally the spot urine should be taken at approximately the same time of day as there is a diurnal variation in protein excretion (reduced at night), whereas the urinary excretion of creatinine is relatively constant.

Patients with heavy proteinuria require measurement of the serum albumin concentration as they may be nephrotic. The presence of proteinuria greater than 1 g per 24 h, microscopic haematuria, impaired renal function, hypertension, or a suggestive clinical or family history increases the likelihood of significant underlying renal pathology; such patients need full investigation. Patients with significant proteinuria benefit from rigorous blood pressure control if hypertensive and treatment with ACE inhibitors (even if normotensive) as these drugs lower the intraglomerular hydrostatic pressure and reduce proteinuria. Nephrotic patients typically have markedly raised cholesterol levels, and cholesterol-lowering treatment such as statin therapy is indicated. Nephrotic patients are also hypercoagulable and should receive prophylaxis for deep vein thrombosis.

Isolated proteinuria

If proteinuria is present only after strenuous exercise or urinary tract infection, or during febrile illnesses, it is likely to be unimportant. Young patients with dipstick proteinuria, however, do require the exclusion of benign orthostatic proteinuria. This condition is characterised by the absence of proteinuria following a period of recumbency: a fresh morning urine sample is negative for protein, with proteinuria becoming detectable later during the day. If patients are collecting a 24-h urine specimen then it is useful to perform a 'split' collection and analyse the early morning urine separately. The long-term prognosis for this condition is very good.

Microscopic haematuria in the absence of proteinuria

Several urine specimens should be analysed in order to ensure that the haematuria is not a transient finding, and urinary tract infection should be excluded. Other potentially confounding factors include menstruation, exercise-induced haematuria (marathon runners!) and the ingestion of various food colourings. Malignancy of the urinary tract and renal stones should be considered in patients over 40 years of age. Relevant investigations include renal ultrasonography and a kidney, ureter and bladder (KUB) X-ray, as well as possible referral to the urologist for a cystoscopy. The presence of a family history of renal disease, hypertension or impaired renal function would merit referral to a nephrologist for a full assessment, to exclude intrinsic renal disease.

When should I check renal function?

The measurement of serum urea, creatinine and electrolytes is common, and often performed as a 'routine test' before surgery. However, it should be considered in many patients, including:

- All patients with microscopic haematuria and/or proteinuria
- All renal transplant patients
- Any seriously ill patient
- Patients with previously documented renal disease as renal function may deteriorate further in the context of an acute illness ('acute on chronic' renal failure)
- Patients receiving potentially nephrotoxic drugs, e.g. aminoglycosides, NSAIDs
- Patients who are oliguric (urine output <400 mL/day)
- Patients commenced on an ACE inhibitor, as initiation of this treatment may result in a deterioration of renal function and/or hyperkalaemia. These complications are more common in patients with diabetes, vascular disease or pre-existing renal impairment as such patients may have occult renovascular disease. Serum urea,

creatinine and electrolytes should be checked before ACE inhibitor treatment and at 4 days (moderate–high risk patients) or 7 days (low risk patients) after commencing the ACE inhibitor. A repeat blood test should be performed at 10 days in moderate–high risk patients and after changes in the dose of ACE inhibitors or diuretics. Note that similar adverse effects may occur with angiotensin receptor blockers. A rise of up to 20% in the serum creatinine level after starting treatment with an ACE inhibitor may be tolerated, but underlying renovascular disease should be considered if the increase is more marked. The ACE inhibitor should be discontinued if the serum potassium level becomes significantly increased.

What do I do with the result?

If the result indicates renal impairment then previous laboratory data are invaluable, even if they have to be obtained from another hospital or the general practitioner. This may indicate whether the renal impairment is acute or chronic, as well as giving an indication of the rate of deterioration. If a number of values for plasma creatinine concentration are available, a reciprocal creatinine plot may be generated; if the slope is steep, this may reinforce the severity of the situation. In addition, patients with a serum creatinine level that is rising 'through the normal range' need a careful assessment as this is also an omen that all is not well.

Patients who develop renal impairment require a thorough and careful clinical assessment as well as scrutiny of the drug chart. Have they received nephrotoxic drugs, such as aminoglycosides (?recent drug levels), NSAIDs or ACE inhibitors? Have they undergone a radiological procedure involving the administration of contrast medium? Important physical signs include evidence of generalised vascular disease with reduced or absent peripheral pulses, bruits, etc. (underlying renovascular disease), skin rashes (allergic interstitial nephritis, vasculitis, endocarditis), fever (sepsis), or a palpable bladder (prostatic obstruction) or kidneys (polycystic kidney disease).

Most acute renal failure that occurs in a hospital setting is secondary to acute tubular necrosis, which may result from severe sepsis, hypotension or renal toxins. In all such patients, a careful assessment of fluid status is critical as the patient may be clinically hypovolaemic (low jugular venous pressure [JVP], postural hypotension, weight loss) and have developed pre-renal uraemia. Potential causes include excessive administration of diuretics, insufficient intravenous fluid replacement, and excessive gastrointestinal (vomiting, diarrhoea) or renal (polyuria secondary to uncontrolled diabetes mellitus or diabetes insipidus) losses. It should be remembered that patients with established chronic renal impairment exhibit a defective capacity to concentrate their urine and are therefore more prone to the development of 'acute on chronic' renal failure. If detected at an early stage 'pre-renal' uraemia is readily remediable by the administration of intravenous fluids, with appropriate monitoring of urine output and blood pressure. Renal function may, however, deteriorate further if pre-renal uraemia is undetected or treated inappropriately, e.g. administration of furosemide to an oliguric patient who is dehydrated.

In contrast, some patients with acute or chronic renal impairment may be salt and water overloaded (raised JVP, hypertension, peripheral oedema, basal pulmonary crepitations), such that further administration of fluids may be dangerous and provoke acute pulmonary oedema. The levels of serum potassium must be monitored closely and drugs that may cause hyperkalaemia discontinued (potassium supplements, potassium-sparing diuretics, etc.).

Differential diagnosis of renal failure

There are myriad causes of renal failure, classically categorised as pre-renal, renal or post-renal. Renal ultrasonography is essential to successful management and provides very important information. If the kidneys are normal in size and non-obstructed, the patient has acute renal failure. The presence of small atrophic kidneys or large cystic kidneys indicates an element of chronic renal impairment. Asymmetry in renal size suggests unilateral congenital dysplasia, renal scarring secondary to reflux nephropathy, or renovascular disease with unilateral ischaemic renal atrophy. However, it is important to note that patients with pre-existing chronic renal failure may develop acute-on-chronic renal failure for any of the reasons outlined previously, and this is potentially reversible if diagnosed and treated appropriately.

Pre-renal causes

- Hypovolaemia, e.g. acute blood loss, third space sequestration of fluid (bowel obstruction), hypotension (systemic sepsis, myocardial infarction)
- Reduction in renal blood flow (e.g. renovascular disease).

Renal causes

Glomerular disease

The differential diagnosis is wide but includes diabetic nephropathy, forms of glomerulonephritis (IgA nephropathy, membranous nephropathy, focal segmental glomerulosclerosis); lupus nephritis, antineutrophil cytoplasmic antibody (ANCA)-positive vasculitis, haemolytic uraemic syndrome.

Tubulointerstitial disease

Acute tubular necrosis is the commonest cause of acute renal failure in hospitalised patients and may be multifactorial in aetiology, for example sepsis, severe hypotension or nephrotoxic drugs (aminoglycosides, NSAIDs). Drug-induced interstitial nephritis may be a complication of myriad drugs including antibiotics and diuretics. Patients with adult polycystic kidney disease have a characteristic appearance on renal ultrasonography. Sarcoidosis may be associated with hypercalcaemia and a raised level of ACE. Patients with analgesic nephropathy typically exhibit small smooth kidneys and have a history of prolonged analgesic intake for arthritis, headaches, etc.

Post-renal causes

There are numerous causes of obstructive nephropathy including prostatic hypertrophy, pelvic malignancy (e.g. cervical carcinoma), retroperitoneal disease (fibrosis, tumour infiltration), transitional cell carcinoma of the ureter, or renal calculi in a single functional kidney. In addition, myeloma may cause acute intra-renal obstruction of nephrons as a result of the intratubular precipitation of filtered light chains ('myeloma kidney').

Management

The aims of management for all patients with acute or chronic renal failure include:

- Actively treat any readily reversible component, e.g. intravenous fluids in patients with pre-renal uraemia, stop nephrotoxic drugs, commence immunosuppression for acute lupus nephritis.
- Minimise the rate of subsequent progression of renal failure, e.g. tight diabetic and blood pressure control, reduce proteinuria with ACE inhibitor treatment.

- Treat and prevent complications, e.g. oral sodium bicarbonate for a metabolic acidosis, vitamin D derivatives for secondary hyperparathyroidism and the prevention of renal bone disease, oral phosphate binders for hyperphosphataemia.
- Modify cardiovascular risk (smoking, lipids) as patients with renal disease exhibit a much higher cardiovascular mortality. This is particularly marked in young patients (<30 years old) who have a 100-fold increase in cardiovascular mortality compared with age-matched controls.
- Make a definitive diagnosis if possible, as treatment may be available and some diseases may recur following renal transplantation, e.g. focal segmental glomerulosclerosis.
- Ensure a smooth transition to renal replacement therapy if and when indicated.

Learning point

When managing patients with renal failure, liaise with senior colleagues at an early stage to ensure optimal early management and prevent potentially serious complications.

Fluid balance

Patients with significant renal impairment have diminished homeostatic mechanisms regarding salt and water balance, and therefore fluid replacement therapy must be appropriate (not too much and not too little). Close monitoring of serum electrolytes is required during such intravenous treatment in order to avoid electrolyte disorders such as hyponatraemia. In general the administration of potassium is avoided as few patients with renal impairment become significantly hypokalaemic, but hyperkalemia is a real risk. In severely ill patients the monitoring of central venous pressure may be a useful guide to fluid treatment.

Renal biopsy

If a patient develops renal failure in the context of unobstructed, normally sized kidneys and the cause is not apparent, a renal biopsy should be considered and the patient discussed with the nephrology team. Such patients also undergo extensive immunological tests as these may be informative, e.g. complement levels, antinuclear antibody, ANCA, antiglomerular basement antibody levels, serum IgG electrophoresis, urinary Bence Jones protein, etc. (see Chapter 10).

Renal replacement therapy

Dialysis is indicated for:

- Hyperkalaemia unresponsive to conventional medical management (see Chapter 2)
- Severe uraemia with a low GFR, especially if the patient has severe nausea, is obtunded or develops uraemic pericarditis
- Severe fluid overload in oliguric patients with severe renal failure who are unresponsive to diuretic therapy.

Current practice is to initiate haemodialysis earlier rather than later in patients in whom it is apparent that the renal failure is irreversible or will require time to respond to treatment. The adjustment of fluid status by dialysis allows appropriate nutritional support and the administration of drugs, blood products, etc. Peritoneal dialysis is not commonly used for patients with acute renal failure but is a useful modality for chronic renal replacement therapy.

CHAPTER 4

Metabolic acid–base disorders

Introduction

Disorders of acid–base balance are commonly encountered in acutely unwell or complicated medical and surgical patients but the interpretation of acid–base data must be placed in the context of the clinical situation in order to be used to maximal effectiveness. In addition, an understanding of some key physiological principles is required.

Acid–base homeostasis

The plasma concentration of hydrogen ion (H^+) is very low ($\sim$40 nmol/L) and is maintained within a very narrow range by:

1. buffering, with excretion of CO_2 by lungs
2. excretion of H^+ by the kidneys.

pH
The pH of a solution is equal to the negative logarithm of the hydrogen ion concentration:

$$pH = -\log[H^+]$$

The pH of extracellular fluid (ECF) is maintained within a narrow range (close to 7.4) which equates to a $[H^+]$ of 40 nmol/L. These tiny concentrations of H^+ can be contrasted to the millimolar concentrations of Na^+ in the ECF (one million times greater) and to the daily load of H^+ (1 mmol/kg) that must be excreted. Venous pH is 0.05 less than arterial pH owing to the generation of carbon dioxide in the tissues before removal by the lungs. In addition, the intracellular pH is lower than extracellular pH and varies between tissues (e.g. skeletal muscle ~7.06, proximal convoluted tubule ~7.13). It is important to note at the outset that nanomolar changes in $[H^+]$ will generate biologically significant changes in pH. For example, a change in $[H^+]$ from 40 to 25 nmol/L will result in a large change in pH from 7.4 to 7.6.

The Henderson–Hasselbalch equation

pH is determined by the ratio of HCO_3 to the partial pressure of carbon dioxide (PCO_2) as given by Henderson–Hasselbalch equation:

$$pH = pKa + \log[base]/[acid]$$

or

$$pH = 6.1 + \log[HCO_3^-]/[H_2CO_3]$$

The H_2CO_3 concentration can be derived from the arterial PCO_2 by multiplying by the solubility constant for CO_2 in plasma (0.03 in mmHg):

$$pH = 6.1 + \log[HCO_3^-]/[0.03 \times PCO_2]$$

In the normal state, the kidneys maintain the $[HCO_3^-]$ at ~24 mmol/L and the lungs maintain the PCO_2 at about 40 mmHg (5.3 kPa).

Where does the acid load come from?

On a normal diet, the metabolism of fats and carbohydrate generates 15000 mmol CO_2 per day, which is excreted by respiration. The metabolism of proteins results in the generation of non-carbonic acids from sulphur-containing amino acids (methionine and cysteine generate H_2SO_4) or non-sulphur-containing amino acids (lysine and arginine generate HCl). In addition, the metabolism of organophosphates yields small amounts of H_3PO_4 and there is a small daily production of acid from cellular metabolism (lactic acid, pyruvic acid, acetic acid). There is also some daily production of alkali from amino acids (glutamate, aspartate) as well as organic anions (acetate, citrate). Vegetarian diets contain higher levels of alkali-containing foods.

> A normal diet generates ~ 1 mmol/kg H^+ per day as non-volatile acids, resulting in a net daily acid load of 50–100 mmol H^+ (1 mmol/kg). These non-volatile acids cannot be excreted by respiration and *must* be excreted by the kidneys.

How does the body deal with the daily acid load?

The daily acid load and maintenance of the extracellular pH close to 7.4 is achieved by three key processes:

1. buffering free H^+ ions
2. alveolar ventilation, which removes CO_2
3. H^+ excretion by the kidneys.

Buffers

A buffer is a substance (usually a weak acid or its base) that is able to release or take up H^+ and is thus able to minimise any changes in H^+ concentration. Buffers are present in both the extracellular (ECF) and intracellular (ICF) fluid compartments. It should be noted that buffers minimise changes in pH but *do not remove acid from the body*.

ECF buffers

HCO_3 is the most important buffer in the ECF. Minor additional buffers include plasma proteins and inorganic phosphates. HCO_3 buffers H^+ to generate water and CO_2 that is excreted by alveolar ventilation:

$$H^+ + HCO_3^- \leftrightarrow H_2CO_3 \leftrightarrow H_2O + CO_2$$

As the level of HCO_3^- falls, the buffering capacity of the ECF falls and the defence against overwhelming acidosis is diminished. Renal excretion of H^+ must occur in order to replenish HCO_3^- buffer.

ICF buffers

These comprise various intracellular proteins (imidazole group on histidines), haemoglobin in erythrocytes, HCO_3^- and phosphates (Table 4.1). Buffering of H^+ in bone by calcium carbonate and calcium phosphates can lead to bone demineralisation. The greater availability of intracellular buffers leads to a more efficient maintenance of intracellular pH.

> The majority of H^+ is buffered initially by bicarbonate in the extracellular fluid. Other buffers are recruited as the acid load increases.

Respiratory control of pH

From the Henderson–Hasselbalch equation we can see that the pH is determined by the PCO_2 and the HCO_3^-. The PCO_2 is controlled by respiratory ventilation and is maintained close to 40 mmHg in the normal resting state. Around 15 000 mmol CO_2 are generated each day from fat and carbohydrate metabolism. The accumulation of CO_2 with the resultant formation of H_2CO_3 is prevented by alveolar ventilation. The increased $[H^+]$ is sensed by medullary chemoreceptors, which signal to the brainstem respiratory centres to increase ventilation.

Hypoventilation therefore results in an accumulation of CO_2, the formation of H_2CO_3, and a respiratory acidosis. Conversely, hyperventilation leads to an excessive removal of CO_2 ('blowing off CO_2') and a respiratory alkalosis (see Respiratory acid–base disorders in Chapter 5).

Table 4.1 Distribution of buffers in a 70-kg man, assuming a total body water of 42 L, [HCO₃]ₑCF of 24 mmol/L and [HCO₃]ᵢCF of 12 mmol/L

Location	Buffers (mmol)			
	HCO_3^-	Protein	Phosphate	Other
ECF	336	<10	<15	0
ICF	336	400	<50	Minor

Renal regulation of pH

The kidneys perform two key functions

1. excretion of acid (mostly as NH_4Cl)
2. regeneration of HCO_3^-.

CO_2 is generated when an acid load is buffered by HCO_3^- and is excreted by alveolar ventilation. Unless the HCO_3^- is regenerated by the kidneys, the HCO_3^- levels will fall and the buffering capacity of the ECF will diminish. This is achieved by:

- Reclamation of all filtered HCO_3^- to avoid simply excreting buffer (Fig. 4.1). This occurs primarily in the proximal tubule and is dependent on brush border carbonic anhydrase, apical Na^+–H^+ antiporter and basolateral Na^+–$3HCO_3^-$ co-transporter. This process is driven by the basolateral Na^+–K^+-ATPase.
- Excretion of H^+ with the resultant generation of HCO_3^- (Fig. 4.2). In a 70-kg man, the daily acid load of 70 mmol H^+ is excreted as 40 mmol NaH_2PO_4 and 30 mmol NH_4Cl. The amount of NaH_2PO_4 is fixed and, to excrete a greater acid load, extra NH_4^+ (ammonium) can be generated and excreted with the resultant generation of more HCO_3^-.

When should I check acid–base balance?

The assessment of acid–base should be considered in:

- Any seriously ill patient, e.g. multiorgan failure, severe pancreatitis
- Patients with respiratory disease and/or respiratory failure
- Patients with uncontrolled diabetes mellitus
- Patients who have, or are suspected of having, ingested drugs or poisons such as ethylene glycol (antifreeze) that can affect acid–base balance.

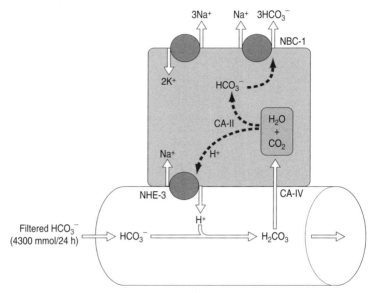

Figure 4.1 Reclamation of filtered HCO_3^-. With a daily glomerular filtration rate of 180 L, approximately 4300 mmol (180 × 24) of HCO_3^- must be reabsorbed. Some 90% of HCO_3^- reabsorption occurs in the proximal convoluted tubule where it is coupled to Na^+ reabsorption. Na^+ is reabsorbed by a sodium hydrogen exchanger (NHE-3) on the apical membrane, driven by a basolateral Na–K-ATPase. The secreted H^+ combines with luminal HCO_3^- in setting of the brush border carbonic anhydrase enzyme (CA-II), producing H_2O and CO_2, which diffuses into the proximal tubular cell. Recombination of intracellular CO_2 with H_2O (catalysed by a different carbonic anhydrase enzyme) produces HCO_3^-, which leaves the cell by a basolateral Na^+–$3HCO_3^-$ co-transporter and enters the circulation. A failure of proximal tubular reabsorption of HCO_3^- results in a proximal renal tubular acidosis. NBC-1, Na^+–HCO_3^- co-transporter

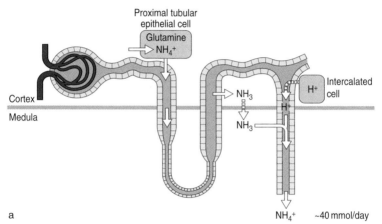

a

NH₄⁺   ~40 mmol/day

Figure 4.2 (a) Excretion of NH_4Cl. H^+ is secreted by the kidney, mostly buffered by ammonia (NH_3). Ammonium (NH_4^+) is generated in proximal tubular cells from glutamate and secreted by the Na^+–H^+ exchanger (NHE-3) into the tubular lumen. The NH_4^+ is reabsorbed by the Na^+–K^+–$2Cl^-$ co-transporter (NH_4^+ replaces K^+) in the ascending loop of Henle and dissociates into NH_3 and H^+; this H^+ is used to reabsorb further HCO_3^-. NH_3 diffuses from the renal medulla into the lumen of the cortical collecting duct, where it buffers H^+ and is excreted as NH_4Cl.

(Continued)

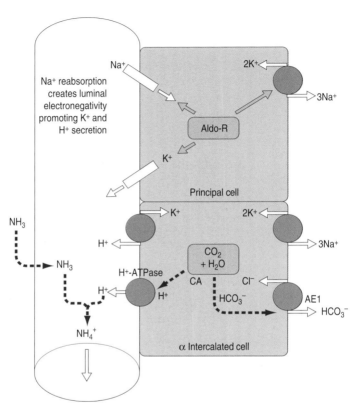

b

Figure 4.2 cont'd (b) Reabsorption of Na$^+$ (promoted by aldosterone) in the principal cells of the cortical collecting duct imparts a negative charge to the tubular lumen, facilitating the secretion of H$^+$ by the H$^+$-ATPase of intercalated cells (secretion of K$^+$ is also promoted). Aldo-R, aldosterone receptor; AE1, anion exchanger 1; CA, carbonic anhydrase. See also Figure 2.2.

Seven steps to the clinical assessment of acid–base status

See Figure 4.3.

Step 1: What is the pH (normal 7.35–7.45)

pH <7.35 implies acidaemia

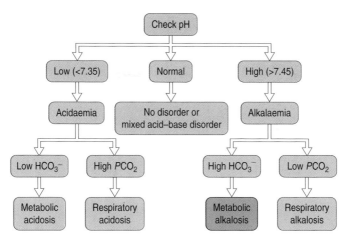

Figure 4.3 Initial assessment of acid–base status. Note that PO_2 has no direct effect on acid–base analysis.

pH >7.45 implies alkalaemia

pH in the normal range implies either no acid–base disturbance or a complex disorder where acidosis and alkalosis exactly cancel each other out.

Step 2: Check the serum bicarbonate (HCO₃) (normal 22–30 mmol/L)

HCO_3 <22 implies metabolic acidosis
HCO_3 >30 implies metabolic alkalosis

Step 3: Check the arterial PCO_2 (normal 35–45 mmHg [4.5–6.0 kPa])

PCO_2 >40 mmHg implies respiratory acidosis
PCO_2 <40 mmHg implies respiratory alkalosis

Step 4: Assess the compensatory responses

In order to maintain the pH within the narrow physiological range, the kidneys try to compensate for respiratory acid–base disorders and the lungs try to compensate for metabolic disorders. For example, in the setting of a metabolic acidosis (low pH, low HCO_3), alveolar ventilation increases, creating a respiratory alkalosis (low PCO_2) in order to return the pH towards the normal range. Similarly, in the

69

setting of a respiratory acidosis (low pH, high PCO_2), the kidneys excrete increased amounts of H^+ and create a metabolic alkalosis (high HCO_3) in order to return the pH toward the normal range.

> Respiratory or metabolic compensation never over-corrects the pH. If the pH is acidaemic (pH <7.4), an acidosis is the primary acid–base disorder, and if the pH is alkalaemic (pH >7.4) then an alkalosis is the primary acid–base disorder.

The degree of compensation can be determined from the equations in Box 4.1. A mixed respiratory metabolic acid–base disorder may be present if the change in PCO_2 is inappropriate for the change in HCO_3 (or vice versa). For example, in a metabolic acidosis with a serum $[HCO_3]$ of 16, you would expect the PCO_2 to drop by ~8 mmHg (1.2 kPa) (see Box 4.1). If the actual PCO_2 has dropped by 20 mmHg, this implies the presence of an additional respiratory alkalosis, i.e. a metabolic acidosis and respiratory alkalosis, as can occur in aspirin intoxication.

Box 4.1 Renal respiratory compensations

Metabolic acidosis

For every 1-mmol/L drop in $[HCO_3^-]$, expect PCO_2 to be reduced by 1 mmHg, from 40 mmHg (0.15 kPa from 5.3 kPa).

Metabolic alkalosis

For every 1-mmol/L rise in $[HCO_3^-]$, expect PCO_2 to be increased by 0.6 mmHg.

Respiratory acidosis

Acute: Expect a 1-mmol/L increase in $[HCO_3^-]$ per 10-mmHg rise in PCO_2.
Chronic: Expect a 3.5-mmol/L increase in $[HCO_3^-]$ per 10-mmHg rise in PCO_2.

Respiratory alkalosis

Acute: Expect a 2-mmol/L decrease in $[HCO_3^-]$ per 10-mmHg fall in PCO_2.
Chronic: Expect a 4-mmol/L decrease in $[HCO_3^-]$ per 10-mmHg fall in PCO_2.

Step 5: Assess the anion gap

The anion gap is the calculated difference between cations and anions in the blood, and is roughly equal to the negative charge contributed by proteins (Fig. 4.4). The anion gap (AG) can be calculated from the equation:

$$AG = (Na^+ + K^+) - (Cl^- + HCO_3^-)$$

which is roughly equal to 16. However, the concentration of K^+ does not vary much (~4 mmol/L), and for convenience the equation becomes:

$$AG = Na^+ - (Cl^- + HCO_3^-) = 12$$

Cations (mmol/L)	Anions (mmol/L)
Sodium 140	Chloride 104
	Bicarbonate 24
Potassium 4.5	Proteins 16 (mEq/L)
Calcium 2.5	Phosphate ~1.2
Magnesium ~1	Sulphate ~1
Others (Fe, Se, Zn, etc.) ~2	Others (organic anions, etc.) ~2–4

Figure 4.4 Cations and anions found in serum. Note that the numbers of each are identical. H^+ is not illustrated as its concentration is in nanomoles, one million times less than the millimolar concentrations depicted. Subtracting the measured anions from the measured cations gives the anion gap, which is roughly equal to the multivalent charge on albumin. As the ions in the shaded area approximately cancel each other out, the anion gap can be calculated from the equation $AG = (Na^+ + K^+) - (Cl^- + HCO_3^-)$. This is often simplified by removing the K^+, as it is the change in the anion gap and not the absolute value that is clinically useful.

te that the normal value for the anion gap is dependent upon the serum protein concentration and approximates to $0.3 \times$ [albumin] (g/L). In a person with a hypoalbuminaemic condition such as the nephrotic syndrome, with a serum albumin concentration of 30 g/L, the expected anion gap would be 9. Although rare, *cationic* proteins, as may be found in patients with myeloma, can result in a falsely increased value for the anion gap.

Causes of a low anion gap

1. hypoalbuminaemia
2. positively charged paraproteinaemia (myeloma)
3. rarely, addition of halides to the serum

The anion gap is calculated for two main reasons.

1. To help determine the aetiology of a metabolic acidosis
2. To determine whether a complex metabolic disorder is present. For example, a diabetic patient with a metabolic ketoacidosis may have a simultaneous metabolic alkalosis secondary to severe vomiting.

Step 6: Assess the (change in serum anion gap/change in HCO_3) (the 'delta/delta')

If HCO_3^- were the only buffer there would be a 1:1 relationship between the increase in anion gap and the fall in serum $[HCO_3^-]$ in a raised anion gap metabolic acidosis. Certainly, with mild degrees of acidosis this is the case, but as the acid load increases the H^+ is buffered by other buffers (predominantly intracellular) and the change in anion gap is usually greater than the change in HCO_3^-.

However, if the delta/delta ratio is much greater than expected (i.e. >1.5:1), this suggests the simultaneous presence of an underlying metabolic alkalosis (which raises the $[HCO_3^-]$) and a raised anion gap metabolic acidosis (e.g. vomiting in patient with diabetic ketoacidosis). Rarely a patient may have a normal $[HCO_3^-]$ and the only clue to the presence of a metabolic acidosis is the raised anion gap value.

Similarly, if the delta/delta ratio is much less than expected (i.e. <1 : 1), this implies the presence of a normal anion gap acidosis in addition to the raised anion gap metabolic acidosis (e.g. a patient with renal tubular acidosis who develops a lactic acidosis).

Step 7: Identify underlying cause of acid–base disturbance

Once the type of acid–base disorder has been identified it is important to establish the underlying cause of the disorder. This requires a careful history, examination, and a variety of biochemical tests. The cause may be obvious if a patient presents with an acute abdomen and has a grossly raised serum amylase level. However, it may be a careful drug history that provides the diagnosis in an elderly diabetic patient with renal impairment who has been commenced on metformin and has developed a lactic acidosis as a complication of this treatment.

Metabolic acidosis

As $[H^+]$ is determined by the ratio of PCO_2 to HCO_3^-, the appropriate respiratory response to a metabolic acidosis ($\downarrow HCO_3^-$) is to hyperventilate ('blow-off CO_2'). The PCO_2 falls by 1 mmHg per 1 mmol drop in HCO_3^-. Patients with a severe metabolic acidosis exhibit a marked increase in ventilation due to both an increased respiratory rate and an increased depth of respiration, and this is described as Kussmaul respiration. The failure to lower PCO_2 by 1 mmol per mmol drop in HCO_3^- implies the presence of a simultaneous respiratory acidosis, i.e. a mixed acid–base disturbance.

A metabolic acidosis is usually present if the serum $[HCO_3^-]$ is less than 22 mmol/L. Rarely, this may be a compensatory response to a chronic respiratory alkalosis (e.g. pregnancy), in which case the pH will be >7.4.

Causes of metabolic acidosis (Fig. 4.5)

A metabolic acidosis can be caused by:
1. a gain of acid, or
2. a loss of HCO_3^-.
Calculation of the anion gap aids in establishing the cause of the metabolic acidosis.

Why does a lactic acidosis cause a raised anion gap, whereas diarrhoea causes a normal anion gap acidosis? Consider adding 5 mmol/L lactic acid to the body. This will be buffered primarily by $NaHCO_3$, resulting

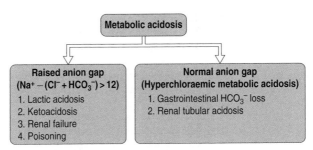

Figure 4.5 Causes of a metabolic acidosis.

in roughly 5 mmol/L sodium lactate and 5 mmol/L H_2CO_3. The $H_2CO_3^-$ dissociates to H_2O and CO_2, which is removed by ventilation. The result is a lowering of the $[HCO_3^-]$ by 5 mmol, the presence of 5 mmol of unmeasured anions (lactate), with no changes in $[Na^+]$ or $[Cl^-]$. From the anion gap equation ($AG = Na^+ - [Cl^- + HCO_3^-]$), the anion gap now becomes 17 (raised by 5mmol, i.e. a raised anion gap). In contrast, diarrhoea results in the loss of $NaHCO_3$ from the gastrointestinal tract. $NaCl$ will be reabsorbed more avidly to maintain extracellular volume, resulting in an increase in serum $[Cl^-]$. This increase in serum $[Cl^-]$ compensates for the fall in HCO_3^-, such that the sum of $[Cl^- + HCO_3^-]$ remains constant. Thus severe diarrhoea results in a hyperchloraemic normal anion gap metabolic acidosis as there is no increase in any unmeasured anions.

How serious is the metabolic acidosis?

This is dependent on a number of factors, including volume status, rate of generation of acid, presence of hypoxia, degree of respiratory compensation and any associated potassium disorders. In general, a metabolic acidosis is becoming extremely dangerous when the pH is <7.2 and/or the serum $[HCO_3^-]$ is in single figures (<10). The consequence may be depressed myocardial contractility and impaired enzyme function.

The treatment of a metabolic acidosis should be aimed at stopping the production of H^+, e.g. insulin treatment in ketoacidosis or oxygen therapy in a patient with a lactic acidosis. In addition, serious threats associated with acidosis must be treated, e.g. haemodialysis in cases of ethylene glycol poisoning. In addition, dangerous potassium abnormalities can be associated with a metabolic acidosis and these need careful management. For example, hypokalaemia in a patient with a renal tubular acidosis can be exacerbated by treatment of the acidosis.

Lactic acidosis

Cellular metabolism requires adenosine triphosphate (ATP) for energy, much of which is produced from carbohydrate metabolism. One mole of glucose can be metabolised by glycolysis, the Krebs cycle and oxidative phosphorylation to produce 36–38 moles of ATP. In the absence of oxygen as an electron receptor, glucose metabolism would stop as nicotine adenine dinucleotide (NAD^+; a co-factor for glycolysis) is converted to NADH. In humans this does not happen as the NADH can be recycled by the conversion of pyruvate to lactic acid by lactate dehydrogenase, thereby regenerating a supply of NAD^+ for glycolysis (Fig. 4.6).

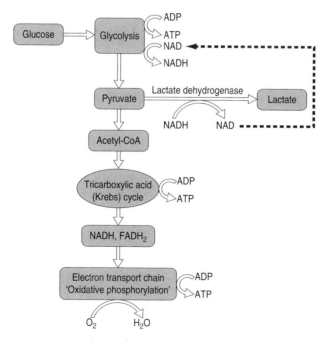

Figure 4.6 Energy production from the metabolism of carbohydrate. In the absence of oxygen, NAD is regenerated by the conversion of pyruvate to lactate, generating a lactic acidosis.

The lactic acid is buffered by serum bicarbonate with the generation of lactate (hence the positive anion gap in lactic acidosis). Normal serum lactate levels are 1–1.5 mmol/L and a lactic acidosis is present if levels are greater than 4–5 mmol/L in an acidaemic patient (Table 4.2). The lactate can subsequently be metabolised by the liver back to pyruvate, and thence to H_2O and CO_2.

Type A lactic acidosis

Clinically any condition that impairs the delivery of oxygen to the tissues will result in the anaerobic metabolism of glucose by glycolysis with the increased formation of lactic acid. This is most often seen in ill patients with hypotension due to sepsis, hypovolaemia or cardiogenic shock. Other causes include prolonged epileptic seizures and carbon monoxide poisoning.

An acute lactic acidosis is commonly seen during marked physical exertion ('the burn') when enhanced energy requirements temporarily outstrip oxygen delivery. An Olympic sprinter can temporarily get their venous pH to ~6.8 with lactate levels greater than 20 mmol/L. However, this is rapidly reversed as the oxygen debt is quickly replaced. However, a critically ill patient in the intensive care unit with sepsis syndrome is likely to have problems with gas exchange and oxygen delivery to tissues from hypotension that are not readily

---

Table 4.2 Causes of a lactic acidosis

Type A	Anaerobic metabolism due to tissue hypoxia
	Shock (hypovolaemic, septic, cardiogenic, anaphylactic)
	Lung problem (severe hypoxaemia <25–30 mmHg)
	Haemoglobin problem (carbon monoxide poisoning)
	Increased oxygen requirement (seizures, sprinting)
Type B	Impaired lactic acid metabolism without hypoxia
	Liver problems with impaired lactate clearance (hepatotoxins, inborn errors, ethanol, tryptophan)
	Mitochondrial disorders → impaired oxidative phosphorylation → increased glycolysis (cyanide, mitochondrial diseases, HIV drugs)
	Impaired pyruvate dehydrogenase (thiamine, inborn errors)
D-Lactic acidosis	Bacterial overgrowth in bowel

reversed even with inotropic support, and is therefore likely to have a persistent metabolic acidosis.

Type B lactic acidosis

A second type of lactic acidosis occurs in patients with abnormal lactate metabolism in the setting of adequate tissue oxygen delivery. This setting is much less common and is usually due to the effect of a drug such as metformin or HIV medications, to inborn errors of metabolism or to mitochondrial dysfunction. It is important to note that metformin is a widely used hypoglycaemic agent which may cause a type B lactic acidosis. This occurs more commonly in those with renal impairment, and this agent should be discontinued when the serum creatinine level climbs above 150 μmol/L or before interventions that may compromise renal function, e.g. intravenous contrast studies.

D-Lactic acidosis

The conditions above refer to the accumulation of the physiological L-form of lactic acid. Rarely in sick patients with bacterial overgrowth in the bowel, gut organisms can produce the isomer D-lactic acid, which cannot be metabolised by the enzyme lactate dehydrogenase as this enzyme only recognizes the L-form. The resulting D-lactic acidosis is important to consider when the cause of a raised anion gap metabolic acidosis is unclear, as D-lactate is not measured by standard assays for lactic acid.

Treatment of lactic acidosis

This is directed at the underlying cause of the lactic acidosis with the aim of increasing tissue oxygenation. Measures to correct shock are the principal intervention. Oxygen therapy may be required in cases of systemic hypoxia. The use of bicarbonate therapy to replace buffer and improve the pH is a controversial issue as it may have deleterious effects. However, $NaHCO_3$ could be considered when the patient is very acidotic, e.g. pH <7.1 or $[HCO_3^-]$ less than 8 mmol/L.

Ketoacidosis

Diabetic ketoacidosis

Diabetic ketoacidosis (DKA) occurs in patients with type 1 diabetes mellitus who have absent or very low levels of insulin. Insulin is required to allow the movement of glucose into most cells (excluding brain and liver) via specific glucose transporters such as GLUT1. This permits glucose metabolism and the production of ATP. In the setting of insulin lack, the serum levels of glucose increase and an alternative source of energy (free fatty acids) is required.

The raised serum glucose concentration raises the serum osmolality, with a resultant shift of water from within cells to the extracellular compartment. An osmotic diuresis occurs with loss of significant amounts of water (~3–6 L), sodium (~600 mmol) and potassium (~200 mmol). The hyperglycaemia is exacerbated by the pre-renal uraemia induced by the osmotic diuresis, as this impairs urinary glucose excretion.

The lack of insulin activates lipolysis in adipocytes with the release of large amounts of free fatty acids (FFAs). The FFAs enter mitochondria where they are oxidised to acetyl-coenzyme A (CoA), which enters the Krebs cycle to produce ATP. When large amounts of acetyl-CoA are produced, they are converted in the liver to ketoacids. These ketoacids can be used as a source of energy, predominantly in the brain and kidneys.

The resultant accumulation of ketoacids (acetoacetic acid and β-hydroxybutyric acid) generates a raised anion gap metabolic acidosis. The volume depletion that accompanies diabetic ketoacidosis may cause sufficient tissue underperfusion to result in a simultaneous lactic acidosis. Although the presence of ketoacids in the urine can be detected by dipsticks, it should be recognised that many dipstick tests for ketoacids do not detect β-hydroxybutyrate, which may be the predominant ketone body. As indicated previously, the degree of increase of the anion gap may be less than expected from the serum [HCO_3^-] (see Step 6, assessment of 'delta/delta'). This may be due to urinary excretion of ketoacids or a concomitant metabolic alkalosis from associated vomiting.

Treatment of diabetic ketoacidosis

Patients with DKA typically present with a decreased level of consciousness, Kussmaul breathing, hyperglycaemia and a severe metabolic acidosis (arterial pH may be less than 7.0). Treatment with intravenous fluids, insulin (typical loading dose of 20 units, then 8–10 units/h intravenously) and potassium replacement will permit correction of the various metabolic abnormalities. Phosphate replacement may also be required. Insulin therapy will allow the metabolism of keto-anions to bicarbonate, which will replenish the buffer. It should be noted that, although a marked acidosis may be present in patients with DKA, the generation of acid from ketogenesis is slow and the rapid correction of the pH with bicarbonate is rarely required and may even be detrimental.

Alcoholic ketoacidosis

Rarely ketoacidosis can occur in patients who are not diabetic. A mild ketosis occurs in starvation. In patients who abuse alcohol, a ketoacidosis may develop – usually in those who have been vomiting and are volume depleted. The insulin deficiency in this setting may be due to intense sympathetic stimulation. Treatment with intravenous fluids alone will reverse the ketoacidosis (dextrose to stimulate insulin release, and saline to replace any volume deficit).

Renal failure

As the number of functioning nephrons decreases, the ability of the kidneys to excrete acid falls. The accumulation of anions such as sulphate, phosphate, urate and hippurate in this setting results in a raised anion gap. The acidosis of renal failure is not usually severe, and typically becomes apparent only when the glomerular filtration rate is <25 mL/min, unless there is a significant normal anion gap acidosis from interstitial diseases such as renal tubular acidosis. The chronic acidosis associated with chronic renal disease, although often mild, is usually treated with oral sodium bicarbonate as it may lead to bone demineralisation and skeletal muscle wasting, and may promote progression of the underlying renal disease.

Poisoning

> Acute poisoning should be considered in patients with a raised anion gap metabolic acidosis and an increased plasma osmolal gap.

Methanol and ethylene glycol

These potentially fatal alcohols are occasionally taken for their intoxicating effects or in a suicide attempt. Metabolism of these compounds by alcohol dehydrogenase produces formic acid (from methanol) or glycolic and oxalic acids (from ethylene glycol), which are responsible for the raised anion gap metabolic acidosis. Clinically, the early signs of intoxication are drunkenness, progressing to coma, nausea, blindness (methanol), oxalate crystalluria and acute renal failure (ethylene glycol), and a raised anion gap metabolic acidosis, which may be severe. Emergency treatment includes inhibiting the metabolism of these alcohols with ethanol, or fomepizole, as this will limit the generation of the toxic metabolites together with haemodialysis.

Osmolal gap

A clue to the presence of these toxins may be made by determining the osmolal gap. This is the difference between the measured plasma osmolality and the calculated osmolality:

$$2 \times [Na] + [glucose] + [urea]$$

The normal value is <10 mOsm, and a high osmolal gap implies the presence of unmeasured osmoles such as alcohol, methanol, ethylene glycol or ketones. An osmolal gap >25 in the setting of a raised anion gap metabolic acidosis is highly suggestive of methanol or ethylene glycol poisoning.

Aspirin

Aspirin intoxication can lead to complex acid–base disturbances. It characteristically results in a respiratory alkalosis from direct stimulation of the respiratory centre, and a mildly raised anion gap metabolic acidosis primarily due to the accumulation of organic acids, lactic acid and ketoacids (not salicylic acid!). Emergency treatment may include alkali therapy and haemodialysis.

Hyperchloraemic metabolic acidosis

> This can generally be regarded as a normal anion gap metabolic acidosis and may be due to gastrointestinal bicarbonate loss or renal tubular acidosis.

Clinical assessment of a hyperchloraemic metabolic acidosis

Once a normal anion gap acidosis has been diagnosed by following steps 1–5 above, it is necessary to try to determine the underlying cause (Fig. 4.7). It is usually relatively straightforward to differentiate between gastrointestinal loss of bicarbonate and renal tubular acidosis from the history of gastrointestinal symptoms. It is, however, more difficult to determine the type of renal tubular acidosis (RTA).

The urine anion gap (UAG)

This is calculated as an estimate of urine ammonium excretion and is derived from the formula:

$$UAG = U_{Na} + U_{K} - U_{Cl}$$

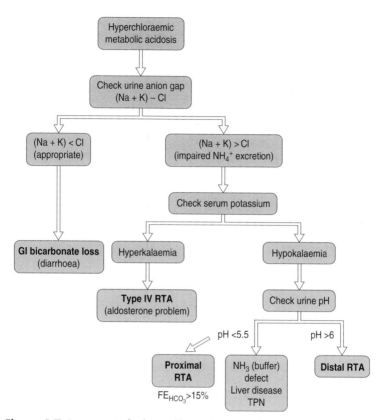

Figure 4.7 Assessment of a hyperchloraemic metabolic acidosis.

The normal value is negative, ranging between −20 and −50 mmol/L, reflecting urine NH_4^+ excretion with Cl^-. In states of metabolic acidosis, the NH_4Cl excretion should increase and the urine anion gap should become progressively more negative (from −75 to −100 mmol/L), reflecting increased excretion of the NH_4^+ cation. However, in RTA there is a failure of ammonium excretion and the UAG has a positive value. This allows differentiation between gastrointestinal HCO_3^- loss and RTA in situations where the history is unreliable. It should be noted that the urine pH may be high in patients with diarrhoea owing to hypokalaemia-induced increased generation of NH_3 and excess buffering of free urinary hydrogen ions.

Gastrointestinal HCO$_3^-$ Loss

Intestinal secretions below the stomach contain a total base concentration of ~60 mmol/L. Diarrhoea can therefore lead to a significant loss of base and a metabolic acidosis. There is no change in the anion gap as unmeasured anions are not added to the serum in these circumstances and there is a concomitant rise in the serum $[Cl^-]$.

As the kidneys can compensate for a metabolic acidosis, the acidosis is rarely marked in this setting unless there is concomitant renal impairment, possibly due to volume depletion. The diminished distal delivery of sodium to the cortical collecting duct (CCD) may also result in impaired renal excretion of potassium and hydrogen ions.

Ureteral diversion into bowel may also generate a normal anion gap metabolic acidosis from HCO_3^-/Cl^- exchange and gut reabsorption of NH_4Cl.

Renal tubular acidosis

> This is due either to the inability to reabsorb filtered bicarbonate (proximal RTA) or to impaired excretion of ammonium chloride (distal RTA).

Proximal RTA

The normal serum concentration of HCO_3^- is 24 mmol/L and the daily glomerular filtration volume is 180 L. This implies that approximately 4300 mmol of HCO_3^- must be reabsorbed by the tubules to prevent loss of buffer in the urine. Some 90% of HCO_3^- reabsorption occurs in the proximal tubule (see Fig. 4.1). Failure to reabsorb HCO_3^- can result in HCO_3^- wasting and a normal anion gap metabolic acidosis (Table 4.3). There may also be an impairment of proximal ammoniagenesis in this condition, resulting in a more positive urine anion gap. Proximal RTA may be isolated but usually occurs in the setting of other evidence of proximal tubular dysfunction such as glucosuria, aminoaciduria and phosphate wasting, and is termed Fanconi's syndrome. The commonest cause of proximal RTA in adults is multiple myeloma.

Table 4.3 Causes of RTA in adults

Proximal RTA

Dysproteinaemias	Multiple myeloma, light chain deposition disease, amyloidosis
Toxins	Heavy metals (lead, mercury, cadmium)
Genetic disorders	Wilson's disease, cystinosis, galactosaemia, hereditary fructose intolerance, Lowe's syndrome, tyrosinaemia
Other	Hyperparathyroidism (hypocalcemia, Vitamin D deficiency), acetazolamide (CA_{II} deficiency), paroxysmal nocturnal haemoglobinuria

Distal RTA

Autoimmune disorders	Sjögren's syndrome, rheumatoid arthritis, SLE, primary biliary cirrhosis
Nephrocalcinosis	Idiopathic hypercalciuria and myriad causes of hypercalcaemia
Drugs	Amphotericin B, ifosfamide, lithium
Interstitial disease	Sickle cell, obstructive uropathy, medullary sponge kidney, renal transplantation
Other	Cirrhosis, myeloma, genetic syndromes (Ehlers–Danlos syndrome, Marfan's syndrome)

In clinical practice, the serum $[HCO_3^-]$ is reset to a new level at which compensatory renal mechanisms are able fully to reabsorb and prevent further loss of HCO_3^- in the urine, i.e. a lowered tubular threshold for HCO_3^- reabsorption. When this is reached, all the filtered HCO_3^- can be reabsorbed and the urine pH becomes appropriately acidic (urine pH <5.5). The typical serum $[HCO_3^-]$ in proximal RTA is 16–18 mmol/L. It is, however, difficult to correct the acidosis as raising the serum $[HCO_3^-]$ leads to an increase of filtered HCO_3^- and wasting of HCO_3^- in the urine. The specific diagnosis of proximal RTA requires the finding of a high urine pH (>7.5) and a high fractional excretion of HCO_3^- (>15%) during HCO_3^- infusion.

Distal RTA

Hydrogen ions are excreted by the kidney predominantly as ammonium chloride (NH_4Cl) and sodium dihydrogen phosphate (NaH_2PO_4). The amount of NaH_2PO_4 is relatively fixed and increased acid loads are excreted predominantly as NH_4Cl. As described in Figure 4.2, excretion of NH_4Cl requires the generation of ammonium from glutamine in the proximal tubule, the medullary recycling of ammonia, the generation of a negative intratubule potential in the CCD, and the secretion of hydrogen ion by the apical H^+-ATPase. Abnormalities in any of these areas can result in a distal RTA (Table 4.4). The commonest cause in adults is Sjögren's syndrome, in which there is reduced expression of H^+-ATPase in the intercalated cells of the CCD.

A more pronounced metabolic acidosis can develop in distal RTA and the serum $[HCO_3^-]$ may fall to less than 10 mmol/L with a urine pH that is always greater than 5.3. However, treatment of the acidosis requires less bicarbonate therapy as the maximum required will be only that necessary to supply sufficient buffer to balance the daily net acid load ($\sim$1 mmol/kg daily). Associated features of distal RTA include hypokalaemia, nephrocalcinosis due to hypercalciuria (bone demineralisation), and hypocitraturia. It is important to note that correction of hypokalaemia should be performed before correction of the acidosis, as correction of the pH will drive potassium into cells and can exacerbate hypokalaemia.

Type IV renal tubular acidosis

Type IV RTA is due to impaired aldosterone secretion or aldosterone resistance, and results in a mild normal anion gap metabolic acidosis in the setting of hyperkalaemia.

Impaired aldosterone action results in impaired Na^+ reabsorption in the CCD and diminished generation of the negative intraluminal potential. This results in failure of H^+ secretion by the intercalated cells in the CCD. There is also a failure of K^+ secretion by the principal cells in the CCD. The hyperkalaemia generates an intracellular acidosis in proximal tubular epithelial cells, and this impairs ammonium generation. The commonest cause of a type IV RTA is the hyporeninaemic hypoaldosteronism that can be found seen in patients with diabetes mellitus. Type IV RTA is usually associated with renal impairment (see Table 4.4). Indeed, patients with advanced diabetic nephropathy develop hyperkalaemia more readily when treated with angiotensin-converting enzyme inhibitors, and may need to start dialysis slightly earlier than non-diabetic patients because of troublesome hyperkalaemia. In patients with type IV RTA the urine pH can often be appropriately lowered to less than 5.3, but the UAG is inappropriately low due to impaired ammoniagenesis.

Table 4.4 Hyperchloraemic (normal anion gap) metabolic acidosis

	Diarrhoea	Proximal RTA	Distal RTA	Type IV RTA
Serum [HCO₃] (mmol/L)	Usually >17	12–20	May be <10	>17
Serum [K] (mmol/L)	Low/normal	Low	Low	High
Urinary pH	Low (rarely high due to ↑NH₃ secondary to hypokalaemia)	<5.5 (in established proximal RTA)	>6	Variable
Urine anion gap [[Na + K] − Cl]	Increased appropriately (Na + K ≪ Cl)	Normal/low (can increase if additional acid load)	Low (impaired NH₄Cl excretion) (Na +K > Cl)	Low (impaired ammoniagenesis) (Na +K > Cl)

Metabolic alkalosis

> A metabolic alkalosis is present if the serum [HCO_3^-] is greater than 30 mmol/L. Rarely this may be a compensatory response to a chronic respiratory acidosis (e.g. chronic respiratory pulmonary disease), in which case the pH will be less than 7.4. A metabolic alkalosis is usually associated with hypokalaemia.

Metabolic alkalosis tends to be a less critical disorder than metabolic acidosis as the generation of alkalosis is usually slow and the kidneys can readily excrete excess HCO_3^-. An impairment of renal excretion is almost always required before a significant metabolic alkalosis can develop. It is important to note that the ability of the proximal tubule to reabsorb HCO_3^- is increased in chronic metabolic alkalosis, and this maintains the alkalosis. This seemingly paradoxical response prevents further loss of Na^+ and HCO_3^- to maintain the extracellular volume.

The lungs compensate for a metabolic alkalosis by hypoventilation, which retains CO_2 and lowers the pH toward the normal range. The PCO_2 should drop by 0.6 mmHg per 1-mmol increase in HCO_3^- (see Box 4.1). Hypokalaemia is almost universally associated with a metabolic alkalosis, and both have similar causes (see Chapter 2). In general, the addition of alkali by itself does not cause a metabolic alkalosis in normal circumstances as the excess base is simply excreted in the urine. However, in the setting of renal impairment the addition of alkali may cause a metabolic alkalosis, as is seen in patients with dyspepsia who develop the milk alkali syndrome.

Causes of metabolic alkalosis (Fig. 4.8)

> Assessment of the volume status is critical to determining the cause of a metabolic alkalosis. The vast majority of metabolic alkaloses are due to vomiting or diuretic use.

The causes of metabolic alkalosis are usually divided into those with a decreased effective arterial blood volume (EABV) and those with an increased EABV. The volume status of the patient is assessed by physical

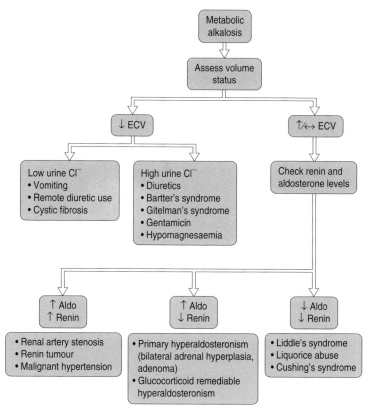

Figure 4.8 Causes of a metabolic alkalosis. Aldo, aldosterone.

examination including the pulse rate, blood pressure, postural changes in blood pressure, presence of oedema, jugular venous pressure, heart sounds, pulmonary crackles, presence of cold peripheries, etc.

Urine electrolytes in metabolic alkalosis

If the kidneys are functioning appropriately, the normal response to a decreased EABV is to retain Na^+, and the urine $[Na^+]$ is typically low

(<20 mmol/L) (Table 4.5). However, in a metabolic alkalosis there may be an obligate loss of Na^+ with HCO_3^- in the urine, and in this setting a more accurate assessment of volume status can be determined from a low urine chloride (<20 mmol/L).

Specific causes of metabolic alkalosis

Vomiting

The concentration of HCl in gastric juice is 125 mmol/L, and several litres may be lost per day with vomiting or nasogastric suction. The associated volume depletion from $NaHCO_3$ loss in the urine leads to an inability of the kidneys to excrete the excess HCO_3^-. In this setting, the urine pH is usually high (>6.0). Note the urine Na^+ may not be as low as predicted in the setting of volume depletion owing to obligate urine loss of Na^+ with HCO_3^-. Treatment with normal saline and KCl will expand the extracellular fluid volume and allow the kidneys to excrete the excess HCO_3^-, thereby correcting the alkalosis.

Diuretics

Diuretic use causes volume depletion due to increased urinary losses of NaCl, and therefore result in secondary hyperaldosteronism. The increased aldosterone concentration, along with the increased delivery of Na^+ to the CCD, results in enhanced reabsorption of Na^+ at this site leading to increased excretion of K^+ and H^+. The hypokalaemia

Table 4.5 Urinary electrolytes in metabolic alkalosis

	Urinary electrolytes (mmol/L)			
	U_{sodium}	$U_{potassium}$	$U_{chloride}$	U_{pH}
Diuretics (recent)	>20	High (>20)	>20	<6.0
Diuretics (remote)	<20	Low (<20)	<20	<5.5
Vomiting (recent)	>20	High (>20)	<20	>7.0
Vomiting (remote)	<20	Low (<20)	<20	<5.5
Bartter's syndrome	>20	High (>20)	>20	6–6.5
Primary hyperaldosteronism[a]	>20	High (>20)	>20	Variable

[a]Extracellular fluid volume is expanded in this condition.

promotes proximal tubule ammoniagenesis, and a metabolic alkalosis results from the excretion of extra NH_4^+. Treatment with NaCl and KCl will allow the kidneys to excrete the excess HCO_3^-.

Other causes of renal salt wasting include interstitial renal disease, an osmotic diuresis or, rarely, Bartter's and Gitelman's syndromes.

Primary hyperaldosteronism

This is also known as Conn's syndrome and is due to either bilateral adrenal hyperplasia or an adrenal tumour (usually an adenoma) producing aldosterone. It typically presents with hypertension with hypokalaemia and a mild metabolic alkalosis. It is a much more common cause of hypertension than is usually appreciated. The mechanism of metabolic alkalosis is similar to that for diuretic use, except the increased distal delivery of Na^+ is due to the volume-expanded state in the setting of aldosterone action. Hypokalaemia is similarly important in augmenting proximal tubule ammoniagenesis.

A good screening test for primary aldosteronism is the aldosterone/renin ratio, which will be high because of a raised aldosterone level and low renin concentration. Treatment consists of antagonism of the aldosterone effects with spironolactone or eplerenone for bilateral adrenal hyperplasia, and surgery if indicated for an aldosterone-secreting adrenal adenoma.

CHAPTER 5

Arterial blood gas analysis

Normal values

See Table 5.1.

Table 5.1 Normal median (range) values for arterial blood gases

Arterial partial pressure of oxygen (PaO_2)	95 (85–100) mmHg
	12.5 (11.0–13.2) kPa
Arterial partial pressure of carbon dioxide ($PaCO_2$)	40 (35–45) mmHg
	5.3 (4.5–6.0) kPa
Standard bicarbonate[a]	24 (22–28) mmol/L

---

[a]Calculated value indicating what the [HCO_3^-] would be at a standard PCO_2 of 40 mmHg (5.3 kPa). The total CO_2 (TCO_2) measured on a serum sample represents the [HCO_3^-] plus the concentrations of dissolved CO_2 and H_2CO_3. It is usually 1–2 mmol/L higher than the [HCO_3^-] value on arterial blood gas analysis.

Oxygen

> Oxygen is required for the production of energy (adenosine triphosphate; ATP) during oxidative metabolism.

Ambient air contains 21% oxygen and the partial pressure of inspired air (PiO_2) at sea-level is 150 mmHg (20 kPa). Gas exchange occurs at the alveolar surface, where the alveolar air is separated from the blood in the pulmonary capillary by a thin layer of capillary endothelial cells, a basement membrane and alveolar epithelial cells lined by surfactant (Fig. 5.1).

Oxygen transport

Oxygen is transported bound to haemoglobin in red cells. Four molecules of O_2 bind per molecule of haemoglobin. The affinity of O_2 for haemoglobin can be reduced by increased levels of 2,3-diphosphoglycerate (2,3-DPG), an increase in $[H^+]$, increased partial pressure of carbon dioxide (PCO_2) and increased temperature. During exercise, the increased $[H^+]$ from lactic acidosis, the increased PCO_2 and the raised temperature all lower the affinity of O_2 for haemoglobin and facilitate O_2 delivery to tissues. 2,3-DPG production is slower, but enhances O_2 tissue delivery in settings such as high altitude and anaemia.

Carbon dioxide

> CO_2 is the end-product of oxidative metabolism of carbohydrates and fats, and is excreted by alveolar ventilation.

CO₂ production

Typically 15 000 mmol CO_2 are produced daily from the metabolism of carbohydrates and fat (~10 mmol/min). During vigorous exercise this can increase to 160 mmol/min.

The CO_2 produced diffuses from cells into red blood cells. Red cell carbonic anhydrase converts this to H^+ and HCO_3^-. The HCO_3^- is

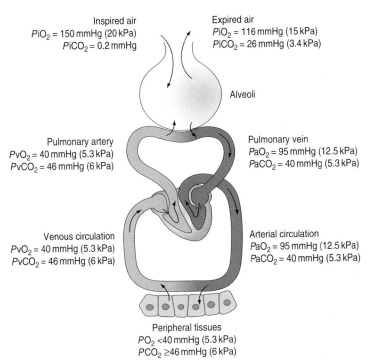

Inspired air
$PiO_2 = 150\,mmHg$ (20 kPa)
$PiCO_2 = 0.2\,mmHg$

Expired air
$PiO_2 = 116\,mmHg$ (15 kPa)
$PiCO_2 = 26\,mmHg$ (3.4 kPa)

Alveoli

Pulmonary artery
$PvO_2 = 40\,mmHg$ (5.3 kPa)
$PvCO_2 = 46\,mmHg$ (6 kPa)

Pulmonary vein
$PaO_2 = 95\,mmHg$ (12.5 kPa)
$PaCO_2 = 40\,mmHg$ (5.3 kPa)

Venous circulation
$PvO_2 = 40\,mmHg$ (5.3 kPa)
$PvCO_2 = 46\,mmHg$ (6 kPa)

Arterial circulation
$PaO_2 = 95\,mmHg$ (12.5 kPa)
$PaCO_2 = 40\,mmHg$ (5.3 kPa)

Peripheral tissues
$PO_2 < 40\,mmHg$ (5.3 kPa)
$PCO_2 \geq 46\,mmHg$ (6 kPa)

Figure 5.1 Gas transport in the pulmonary and systemic circulation. Note that the oxygenated blood in the pulmonary vein is the same as arterial blood in the systemic circulation.

transported into plasma in exchange for chloride (chloride shift) and the H^+ is buffered by haemoglobin. At the lung this process is reversed; CO_2 is released and excreted by alveolar ventilation.

Respiratory function

Control of ventilation

The normal alveolar ventilation is 5 L/min and is controlled by respiratory centres in the brainstem (medulla and pons). Sensory input from receptors for CO_2, H^+ and O_2 modify the standard ventilatory response:

- Central chemoreceptors (ventral surface medulla) stimulate ventilation in response to an increased PCO_2 or decreased pH of the cerebrospinal fluid.
- Peripheral chemoreceptors in the carotid body (type 1 glomus cells) are responsible for the ventilatory response to low arterial partial pressure of oxygen (PaO_2).
- Pulmonary mechanoreceptors respond to local mechanical and chemical stimuli, and may control ventilatory rate.

Lung perfusion

This is equal to the cardiac output (heart rate × stroke volume of right ventricle) and is 5 L/min in an average resting human adult. Oxygen receptors in the pulmonary vasculature may initiate vasoconstriction in response to hypoxia, leading to changes in lung perfusion and ventilation/perfusion (V/Q) matching.

Areas of ventilated lung may be underperfused by a reduction in cardiac output or by regional decreases in perfusion (e.g. pulmonary embolism) leading to hypoxia from V/Q mismatch. By contrast, areas of unventilated lung may be perfused wastefully, resulting in shunting.

Diffusion

Oxygen diffuses from the alveolar air across the alveolar epithelium (covered by surfactant), basement membrane and pulmonary capillary endothelium, and is taken up by haemoglobin. Diffuse lung fibrosis may impair oxygen diffusion. Gas exchange may be assessed by the carbon monoxide transfer factor (T_LCO_2)

Assessment of oxygenation

Clinical assessment

A full clinical examination should be performed with particular emphasis on cardiac and respiratory systems. Cyanosis does not occur until there is 5 g/L deoxyhaemoglobin or an arterial oxygen saturation (SaO_2) of less than 67%. Cyanosis is affected by skin colour, pigmentation and haematocrit. Ventilation should be assessed by examining rate and depth of respiration.

Arterial partial pressure of oxygen (PaO$_2$)

This is measured on arterial blood gas analysis. Normal values on room air are 83–100 mmHg (11–13.2 kPa). Analysis of PaO_2 will identify hypoxaemia, but will not identify the cause, which must be determined from assessment of $PaCO_2$, the alveolar-arterial gradient and other investigations.

Arterial oxygen saturation (SaO$_2$)

SaO_2 assesses oxygenation but not respiratory ventilation. Because of the shape of the oxygen dissociation curve, a small drop in SaO_2 represents a large drop in PaO_2.

This is measured by a pulse oximeter, and in many places has become part of the standard nursing observations.

There are two main pitfalls:

1. SaO_2 gives no information about respiratory ventilation. A low SaO_2 demonstrates hypoxia, but does not determine whether the cause is hypoventilation (e.g. opioids) or another effect. An assessment of ventilation, ideally by arterial blood gas analysis, should be performed in this setting.
2. A large fall in PaO_2 may cause only a small fall in SaO_2 owing to the shape of the oxygen dissociation curve. It is important to recognise that SaO_2 values of 93–95% may reflect a substantial fall in PaO_2 (Fig. 5.2).

Alveolar-arterial oxygen gradient (AA gradient)

This calculation is used in the assessment of hypoxia to determine the contribution of hypoventilation to the decrease in PO_2. It can be followed serially to determine whether a condition is improving or worsening:

AA gradient = 150 mmHg − [(1.25 × $PaCO_2$) + PaO_2]

AA gradient = 20 kPa − [(1.25 × $PaCO_2$) + PaO_2]

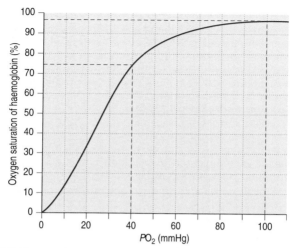

Figure 5.2 Oxygen dissociation curve. Note that the curve is relatively flat down to a PaO_2 of 60 mmHg (8 kPa) and that relatively large changes in PaO_2 can occur without major changes in SaO_2.

Normal values for the AA gradient are 5–10 mmHg (1–1.5 kPa). Hypoventilation will lower the arterial PO_2 but will not increase the AA gradient. By contrast, any impairment of diffusion, V/Q mismatch or shunting will lead to an increased AA gradient.

Notes:

1. The AA gradient can be calculated only when the PO_2 of inspired air is known precisely (i.e. at room air or on a mechanical ventilator (when PaO_2 becomes the FiO_2 [inspired oxygen fraction] $\times$ 713 mmHg).
2. The normal AA gradient increases with age and with increasing FiO_2.

Assessment of tissue hypoxia

Although we are measuring the degree of oxygenation of the blood and the adequacy of ventilation using arterial blood gas analysis, it should be appreciated that these are surrogate values and that what we are most interested in is the adequacy of tissue oxygenation.

Tissue hypoxia is often assessed in ill patients in the intensive care setting. This is done clinically by looking for evidence of organ dysfunction (e.g. hypotension, cold peripheries, adult respiratory distress syndrome [ARDS], acute renal failure, mental obtundation). Other methods include looking for the products of anaerobic metabolism (e.g. serum lactate), assessing the mixed venous oxygen saturation (SvO_2), measuring the ratio of oxygen delivery to oxygen consumption (DO_2/VO_2 ratio) or, rarely, gastric tonometry.

Assessment of ventilation

> Examination of the $PaCO_2$ allows an assessment of alveolar ventilation.

This can be assessed clinically by observing the rate and depth of respiration, although this is inaccurate. Alveolar ventilation is best assessed by measuring the $PaCO_2$. The normal $PaCO_2$ at rest is 40 mmHg (5.3 kPa).

- Increased ventilation will lower the $PaCO_2$ and lead to a respiratory alkalosis.
- Decreased ventilation will raise the $PaCO_2$ and lead to a respiratory acidosis.

Respiratory failure

This is a term used to describe hypoxaemia when PaO_2 is <60 mmHg (8.0 kPa), and is divided into two types:

- Type I respiratory failure is hypoxaemia in the absence of hypercapnia (due to diffusion impairment, shunting or V/Q mismatch (e.g. pulmonary oedema, lung fibrosis, pulmonary embolism, asthma).
- Type II respiratory failure is hypoxaemia in the setting of hypercapnia indicating hypoventilation (e.g. chronic obstructive pulmonary disease [COPD], opioid overdose).

Treatment of hypoxaemia

The underlying cause of hypoxia should be determined and treated (e.g. naloxone treatment for opioid overdose).

Oxygen therapy

Oxygen therapy should be initially prescribed by mask and titrated upwards to achieve SaO_2 >95% (Table 5.2). It should be noted that with most masks the maximum FiO_2 may reach only 35–40%. In order to increase FiO_2 further, 'tusks' or a rebreathing bag may be added to the mask. If oxygenation is still insufficient, consideration should be given to continuous positive airway pressure (CPAP) or mechanical ventilation.

Use of oxygen in patients with chronic respiratory acidosis

In a subset of patients with chronic hypoxia and hypercapnia, oxygen therapy may worsen hypercapnia. The pathophysiology is unclear, but factors include diminished hypoxic ventilatory drive, worsening of V/Q mismatching and decreased affinity of haemoglobin for CO_2. Concern over this feature has led to the inappropriate withholding

Table 5.2 Maximum oxygen delivery by nasal cannulae and mask[a]

	Oxygen flow rate (L/min)	% O_2 delivered
Nasal cannulae	1	24
	2	28
	3	32
	4	36
	5	40
	6 (max)	44
Basic oxygen mask	5–6	40
	6–7	50
	7–8 (max)	60
Mask with reservoir bag (one-way valve on reservoir)	5–8 L	80–85

[a]Patients with a high minute ventilation usually entrain large amounts of room air and markedly dilute the actual concentration of O_2 inspired.

of oxygen from some patients and potential complications from hypoxaemia. In these patients oxygen therapy should be prescribed to maintain a PaO_2 of 60–70 mmHg (8–9 kPa; SaO_2 >90%) and the $PaCO_2$ followed. Problems with respiratory acidosis are unlikely unless the $PaCO_2$ climbs above 80–85 mmHg (10 kPa).

Respiratory acid–base disorders

Respiratory acid base disorders are due to abnormalities of pulmonary ventilation. Hypoventilation leads to a respiratory acidosis and hyperventilation leads to a respiratory alkalosis.

Assessment of respiratory acid–base status

Determination of the acid–base status should be performed according to the seven steps outlined in Chapter 4.

Seven steps for assessing acid–base status

1. Assess the pH.
2. Check the serum HCO_3 level.
3. Check the arterial PCO_2.
4. Assess the compensatory responses.
5. Calculate the serum anion gap.
6. Calculate the delta/delta.
7. Identify the underlying causes.

An arterial blood gas will give the values for pH, arterial PCO_2 and bicarbonate. Similar information can be gained from a venous blood gas, although PCO_2 is typically a little higher (~46 mmHg [6 kPa]) and the venous pH is ~7.35. Of course, the PO_2 will be much lower (~40 mmHg [5.3 kPa]).

Initial assessment of acid–base status (steps 1–3) is shown in Figure 5.3. Although the PCO_2 will allow assessment of alveolar ventilation, it is still necessary to complete all seven steps to interpret the results fully and to avoid missing a complex acid–base disorder (see Chapter 4).

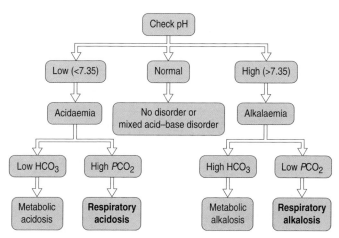

Figure 5.3 Initial assessment of respiratory acid–base disorder.

Is a respiratory acid–base disorder present?

The normal arterial PCO_2 is 40 mmHg (5.3 kPa). A normal $PaCO_2$ with a normal pH (7.4) indicates that there is no respiratory acid–base disorder present.

- An arterial PCO_2 <40 mmHg with pH >7.4 implies a respiratory alkalosis.
- An arterial PCO_2 >40 mmHg, with pH <7.4 implies a respiratory alkalosis.

Is this merely respiratory compensation for a metabolic disorder?

In metabolic acid–base disorders, the change in pH will either stimulate or inhibit respiration in an attempt to return the pH toward normal (7.4). The expected change in PCO_2 for metabolic disorders is shown in Box 5.1.

With a metabolic acidosis, pulmonary *hyper*ventilation would be expected to 'blow off' CO_2; this will partially correct the pH. In this setting the arterial PCO_2 will be low (this is considered normal respiratory compensation or an appropriate respiratory alkalosis).

However, if the degree of hyperventilation is greater than expected, there may be an additional respiratory alkalosis in excess of the

Table 5.3 Examples of arterial blood gases in different conditions

	PaO_2 (mmHg)	$PaCO_2$ (mmHg)	Serum [HCO$_3$] (mmol/L)	pH	AA gradient (mmHg)
Normal	100	40	24	7.4	10
Opioid overdose (acute respiratory acidosis)	70	75	24	7.13	10
COPD (chronic respiratory acidosis)	60	75	35	7.29	25[a]
Anxiety (acute respiratory alkalosis)	110	25	24	7.6	10
Pulmonary fibrosis (chronic respiratory alkalosis)	50	30	20	7.45	75
Oxygen mask[b]	135	40	24	7.4	?

Note the more extreme changes in pH in the acute respiratory disorders due to lack of renal compensation.
[a]V/Q mismatch is often present in COPD (in addition to pure hypoventilation), leading to a raised AA gradient.
[b]Note that $PO_2 + PCO_2 > 150$ mmHg (room air inspired PO_2) implies the patient is receiving supplemental oxygen; in this setting the AA gradient cannot be calculated.

expected compensatory response (as seen in salicylate intoxication). By contrast, if the expected fall is less than expected, a respiratory acidosis is present (e.g. impaired ventilation secondary to narcotics).

Example:

Arterial blood gases reveal pH 7.35, HCO$_3$ 14 mmol/L and PCO_2 26 mmHg.

The low pH and low HCO$_3$ tell us that the primary disorder is a metabolic acidosis. The PCO_2 is low, however, as we would expect the PCO_2 to drop by only 1–1.2 mmHg (from 40 mmHg) for each 1-mmol/L drop in HCO$_3$. This suggests that hyperventilation in excess of the normal compensatory mechanisms is present.

Box 5.1 Respiratory–renal compensation

Metabolic acidosis

For every 1-mmol/L drop in [HCO$_3$], expect PCO_2 to be reduced by 1 mmHg (0.15 kPa) from normal.

Metabolic alkalosis

For every 1-mmol/L rise in [HCO$_3$], expect PCO_2 to be increased by 0.6 mmHg (0.8 kPa) from normal.

Respiratory acidosis

Acute: Expect a 1-mmol/L increase in [HCO$_3$] per 10-mmHg (1.5-kPa) rise in PCO_2.

Chronic (>5 days): Expect a 3.5-mmol/L increase in [HCO$_3$] per 10-mmHg (1.5-kPa) rise in PCO_2.

Respiratory alkalosis

Acute: Expect a 2-mmol/L decrease in [HCO$_3$] per 10-mmHg (1.5-kPa) fall in PCO_2.

Chronic (>3 days): Expect a 4-mmol/L decrease in [HCO$_3$] per 10-mmHg (1.5-kPa) fall in PCO_2.

Renal compensation for a respiratory disorder

In a similar manner to respiratory compensation, the kidneys will try to correct the pH toward normal if there is a respiratory acid–base disorder. This compensation is less efficient than the lungs and takes several days for the maximal change in HCO$_3^-$.

With a respiratory acidosis the kidneys will increase ammonium (NH$_4^+$) excretion to raise serum HCO$_3^-$ concentration, and with a respiratory alkalosis the kidneys will decrease HCO$_3^-$ reabsorption to decrease the serum HCO$_3^-$ level.

The degree to which the HCO$_3^-$ level should change with respiratory acid–base disorders is shown in Box 5.1.

Respiratory acidosis

A respiratory acidosis is due to CO$_2$ retention as a result of hypoventilation.

Carbonic acid (H_2CO_3) cannot be buffered by bicarbonate and the serum HCO_3^- level does not fall with a respiratory acidosis. By contrast, the HCO_3^- concentration rises as the kidney compensates for the respiratory acidosis by increasing ammonium (NH_4^+) excretion. The expected increase is given in Box 5.1.

Example:

Arterial blood gases reveal pH 7.2, HCO_3 16 mmol/L, PCO_2 40 mmHg.

The low pH and low HCO_3 tell us that the primary disorder is a metabolic acidosis. The expected PCO_2 would be ~32 mmHg (see Box 5.1); however, the PCO_2 is higher than expected at 40 mmHg, implying a problem with ventilation. *A respiratory acidosis can therefore be present with a normal PCO_2.*

Clinical features

Acute respiratory acidosis is usually associated with a decreased respiratory rate and often with a decreased level of consciousness. When severe, it may be associated with hypotension.

Chronic respiratory acidosis is often dominated by the associated features of hypoxaemia. Hypercapnia may lead to peripheral vasodilatation with bounding pulse and headache, tachycardia, papilloedema and flapping tremor.

Causes of respiratory acidosis

See Table 5.4.

- The commonest cause of acute respiratory acidosis is central respiratory depression due to drugs (especially opioids), and should be considered in any patient with a reduced respiratory rate.
- Chronic obstructive pulmonary disease is the commonest cause of chronic respiratory acidosis.

Note that the change in serum HCO_3^- may help to differentiate between an acute condition (e.g. drug overdose) and a chronic condition where maximal renal compensation should have occurred (e.g. COPD).

Acute versus chronic respiratory acidosis

In acute respiratory acid–base disorders there has not been time for renal compensation to vary NH_4^+ excretion, and changes in arterial

---

Table 5.4 Causes of respiratory acidosis

Central causes	Central sleep apnoea, cerebral injury or hypoxia, brainstem herniation, status epilepticus, primary hypoventilation
Drugs	Opioids, sedatives, psychotropics, muscle relaxants
Upper airway obstruction	Laryngeal oedema or bronchospasm
Lung problems	Chronic obstructive pulmonary disease (COPD)
Neuromuscular problems	Myasthenia gravis, myotonic dystrophy, trauma

---

pH may be marked. By contrast, chronic respiratory acidosis is tolerated much better due to renal ammonium excretion raising the serum $[HCO_3^-]$. Maximum renal compensation probably occurs by 5–6 days.

Example:

Consider an acute respiratory acidosis in which the PCO_2 rises from 40 to 80 mmHg in a short period. There will be little time for the kidneys to increase ammonium excretion and, from the Henderson–Hasselbalch equation, the pH will go from 7.4 to 6.1 $+ \log(24/0.03 \times 80) = 7.1$. However, in chronic acidosis the kidneys would be expected to raise the serum $[HCO_3]$ by 3.5 mmol per 10-mmHg rise in PCO_2. The new $[HCO_3]$ would be 38 mmol/L and the new pH $(6.1 + \log[38/0.03 \times 80]) = 7.3$.

Treatment of respiratory acidosis

Treatment is aimed at the underlying aetiology of the hypoventilation. Acute respiratory centre depression by opioids may be reversed with naloxone. Upper airways should be cleared or a tracheostomy may be required. Patients with COPD may require bronchodilators and steroids. If the hypoventilation does not respond to these measures, mechanical ventilation may be required.

Respiratory alkalosis

This is a common abnormality due to hyperventilation ('blowing off' CO_2). The significance of this acid–base disorder usually relates to the underlying aetiology.

The kidney compensates for a respiratory alkalosis by increasing urine bicarbonate excretion, creating a compensatory metabolic acidosis. This process occurs rapidly and is usually complete within 48 h. The expected change in serum $[HCO_3^-]$ is given in Box 5.1.

Clinical features

Hyperventilation may be clinically apparent (tachypnoea, Kussmaul respiration). Symptomatically patients may complain of muscle cramps, tingling and paraesthesias. This is due to the alkalosis (low serum $[H^+]$), which promotes increased binding of calcium to proteins, resulting in a decrease in ionised calcium concentration.

Table 5.5 Causes of respiratory alkalosis

Hypoxia	Lung disease, heart failure, altitude, anaemia
Pulmonary receptor stimulation	Lung disease (e.g. pneumonia, pulmonary embolism, pulmonary oedema)
Drugs	Aspirin, theophylline, catecholamines
CNS disorders	Subarachnoid haemorrhage, cerebral injury
Miscellaneous	Anxiety, pregnancy, sepsis, cirrhosis, pain

Causes of respiratory alkalosis

Respiratory alkalosis may be due to stimulation of peripheral chemoreceptors by hypoxia or hypotension, to stimulation of central chemoreceptors by a fall in pH, or to intrinsic pulmonary disease affecting pulmonary receptors (Table 5.5).

Treatment of respiratory alkalosis

Treatment is aimed at the underlying cause of the disorder. Rebreathing of expired air is rarely required.

CHAPTER 6

Calcium, phosphate and magnesium metabolism

Calcium homeostasis

Although calcium levels are measured in the blood, 99% of total body calcium is contained within the mineral content of bones. Serum calcium levels are determined by the balance of calcium entering the blood (following absorption from the gut or resorption from bones) and that leaving the blood (by renal excretion or being utilised during bone mineralisation). During periods of active growth, such as in childhood, there is a net positive balance of calcium. In normal adults the serum calcium levels are generally constant with net calcium input matching output, although elderly patients and postmenopausal women may develop a negative calcium balance.

Extracellular calcium exists in the blood as three forms:

- 45% of total calcium is ionised calcium (the most important physiologically)
- 45% is bound to plasma proteins (principally albumin)
- 10% forms complexes with other molecules (e.g. citrate).

Free ionised calcium is critical in a number of important physiological processes, including nerve conduction, muscle contraction and activation of clotting factors.

Intracellular calcium levels ($\sim$0.001 mmol/L) are markedly lower than extracellular calcium levels (2.2–2.6 mmol/L), so that a large concentration gradient is constantly maintained across the cell membrane. Calcium plays a critical role in many intracellular processes such as cell signalling, contraction, activation and secretory activity. An increase in intracellular calcium concentration may result from the entry of calcium from the extracellular fluid via calcium channels in the plasma membrane, or via release from intracellular calcium stores (mitochondria, sarcoplasmic reticulum).

Regulation of calcium homeostasis

The free ionised calcium level is controlled predominantly by the actions of parathyroid hormone (PTH) and 1,25-dihydroxycholecalciferol (1,25-DHCC, or calcitriol) (Fig. 6.1), with other factors such as calcitonin, oestrogens and glucocorticoids playing a minor role.

Parathyroid hormone

PTH is secreted by the parathyroid glands. PTH secretion is regulated by the interaction between free ionised calcium and the cell surface calcium-sensing receptors (CaR_G) of parathyroid gland cells. PTH secretion is inhibited by hypercalcaemia and stimulated by hypocalcaemia. PTH acts to:

1. increase calcium release from bones by promoting osteoclastic bone resorption
2. stimulate 1α-hydroxylation of vitamin D in the kidney, leading to increased gut absorption of calcium (and phosphate)
3. increase renal tubular calcium reabsorption (and inhibit renal phosphate reabsorption).

Vitamin D

1,25-DHCC is the most active metabolite of vitamin D. Vitamins D_2 and D_3 are present in the diet (e.g. fish oil, plants) and are generated in the skin by the action of ultraviolet light (Fig. 6.2). Conversion to 25-hydroxycholecalciferol by the 25-hydroxylase enzyme occurs in the liver, and this is further converted to 1,25-DHCC by the 1α-hydroxylase enzyme in the kidney (see Fig. 6.2). 1,25-DHCC increases calcium absorption

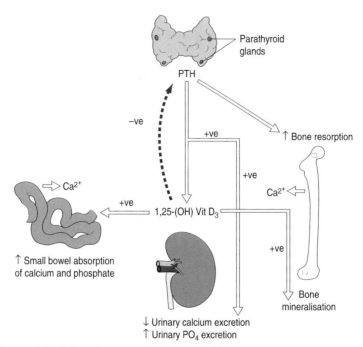

Figure 6.1 Calcium homeostasis. In settings of low serum calcium concentration, PTH is stimulated, resulting in increased calcium release from bone and decreased renal calcium excretion. PTH also stimulates 1α-hydroxylase activity with increased production of 1,25-dihydroxycholecalciferol, which acts to increase gut absorption.

in the intestine by inducing the synthesis of the calcium binding protein, calbindin D_{9k}, in the gut. The kidney also contains a 24-hydroxlase that produces the vitamin D metabolite 24,25-DHCC, which has a less clear function.

Calcitonin

Calcitonin is produced by the parafollicular cells of the thyroid gland. Although calcitonin can reduce serum calcium levels by inhibiting calcium release from bone and renal calcium reabsorption, it has a

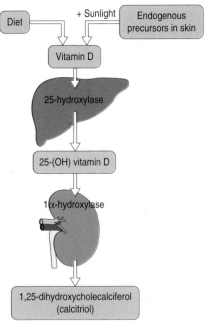

Figure 6.2 Vitamin D metabolism. Vitamin D produced in the skin is 25-hydroxylated in the liver, then 1α-hydroxylated in the kidney to 1,25-dihydroxy-vitamin D (the most active form of vitamin D).

limited action. A chronic increase or deficiency of calcitonin appears to have no clinically relevant effects upon calcium homeostasis or bone mineralisation. Calcitonin levels are, however, useful as a tumour marker in patients with medullary carcinoma of the thyroid.

Assessment of serum calcium levels

Although the *total* serum calcium level is measured in the blood (normal range 2.1–2.6 mmol/L), it is the *ionised* fraction that is important physiologically. There are two settings where the total calcium level may not accurately reflect the ionised calcium concentration.

1. Protein binding

As albumin is the major calcium binding protein in the blood, total calcium levels can be markedly affected by a change in the albumin concentration. Low serum albumin levels will lead to a low total serum calcium level, but the ionised calcium level may still be in the normal range. As a result, the total serum calcium concentration must be 'corrected' for the albumin concentration. In general, the serum calcium falls by 0.02 mmol/L for each 1 g/L fall in serum albumin concentration. A formula commonly used to correct for variation in plasma albumin is:

$$\text{Corrected [calcium]} = \text{Measured [calcium]} + 0.02 \times (40 - \text{[albumin]})$$

Rarely an abnormal monoclonal protein in myeloma will bind calcium and give a raised total, but normal ionised, calcium level.

2. Acid–base status

The level of ionised calcium is affected by the blood pH. Acidosis reduces the ability of albumin to bind calcium, thus resulting in an increase in ionised calcium. An alkalosis induces the opposite effect with a resultant fall in ionised calcium levels. This may be clinically evident in patients who hyperventilate and develop an acute respiratory alkalosis. They may complain of circumoral paraesthesia and may even develop tetany as a result of the acute reduction in ionised calcium. Similarly, in patients who are acidotic, rapid correction of pH with sodium bicarbonate or dialysis may acutely lower the ionised calcium fraction.

When should I consider checking a patient's calcium level?

Consider in patients with:

- neurological symptoms (confusion, irritability, tetany or seizures)
- renal calculi or evidence of abnormal calcification
- suspected or confirmed malignant disease
- polyuria and polydipsia
- drug treatment that can induce hypercalcaemia (e.g. vitamin D derivatives, calcium-containing phosphate binders, thiazide diuretics)
- acute or chronic renal failure

- conditions such as sarcoidosis, thyrotoxicosis that may be complicated by hypercalcaemia
- bone disease (such as rickets or osteomalacia)
- suspected pancreatitis or rhabdomyolysis (both may result in hypocalcaemia).

Hypercalcaemia

Hypercalcaemia should be confirmed with a repeat sample, preferably taken without the use of a tourniquet. Hypercalcaemia is often asymptomatic until levels reach >3 mmol/L. Indeed, many patients with primary hyperparathyroidism are detected incidentally following a 'routine' blood test when they are found to have moderate hypercalcaemia. The symptoms of hypercalcaemia depend upon both the absolute levels and the rate of increase. Marked hypercalcaemia can produce a variety of locomotor, gastrointestinal, renal and even psychiatric symptoms ('bones, stones and abdominal groans'). The commonest causes of hypercalcaemia are hyperparathyroidism and malignant disease (Table 6.1).

Symptoms of hypercalcaemia

- Anorexia, nausea, vomiting, constipation
- Volume depletion
- Polyuria and polydipsia (secondary to antidiuretic hormone antagonism)
- Fatigue
- Mental changes including confusion, depression and psychosis
- Renal stones and nephrocalcinosis
- Pancreatitis

Hyperparathyroidism

Most modern PTH immunoassays measure intact PTH molecules (PTH_{1-84}). Therefore, the PTH-like proteins (PTH_{RP}) produced by some malignant tumours may not be detected using these methods.

Primary hyperparathyroidism

Primary hyperparathyroidism accounts for 10–20% of patients with hypercalcaemia and is usually secondary to a solitary adenoma

Table 6.1 Causes of hypercalcaemia

Hyperparathyroidism	Primary (mostly single adenoma)
	Tertiary (usually secondary to chronic kidney disease)
Malignancy	Solid tumours (may result from metastatic bony invasion, osteoclast activation or release of PTH-related protein)
	Multiple myeloma
Granulomatous disorders	Sarcoid, tuberculosis, leprosy, others
Drugs	Calcium supplements, vitamin D, thiazide diuretics, lithium, theophylline, vitamin A excess
Endocrine	Hyperthyroidism, acromegaly, phaeochromocytoma, multiple endocrine neoplasia (MEN) syndromes, Addison's disease
Other	Prolonged immobility, familial hypocalciuric hypercalcaemia

(80%), diffuse hyperplasia of all four glands (15%) and rarely the result of carcinoma. The typical clinical picture includes a raised PTH level in the context of hypercalcaemia (*note*: the PTH level should be suppressed in these circumstances!). A reduced phosphate level secondary to increased renal phosphate excretion and a raised bony alkaline phosphatase level reflecting increased bone turnover may also be found. In severe cases renal function may be impaired, and radiography may reveal bony changes such as subperiosteal erosion of the phalanges or a 'pepper-pot skull'.

Secondary and tertiary hyperparathyroidism

Patients with chronic renal failure may develop secondary hyperparathyroidism. This reflects an appropriate physiological response to the persistent hyperphosphataemia and hypocalcaemia that accompanies chronic renal failure. Treatment is aimed at reducing plasma phosphate levels with dietary phosphate restriction and phosphate binders (such as calcium acetate, calcium carbonate or sevelamer). These are taken with food and bind phosphate in the gut, preventing phosphate absorption. In addition, treatment with 1α-calcidol or calcitriol will restore 1,25-DHCC levels, promote calcium absorption from the gut and directly inhibit PTH secretion. Patients are monitored by regular checks of calcium, phosphate and PTH levels. However, if secondary hyperparathyroidism is not adequately controlled, patients may develop tertiary hyperparathyroidism characterised by autonomous PTH secretion. Such patients may require surgical intervention.

Hypercalcaemia and malignancy

This is typically due to increased bone resorption from osteolytic metastases (commonly breast and lung cancer) or from tumour secretion of a peptide with PTH activity, called PTH-related protein (PTHrP). Hypercalcaemia is often prominent in multiple myeloma (partly due to the production of osteoclast activating factors), and hypercalcaemia in lymphoma may be secondary to tumour secretion of calcitriol. Of note, by the time hypercalcaemia develops, the tumour is typically advanced and readily apparent.

Granulomatous disorders

Hypercalcaemia may be found in sarcoidosis, and less commonly other granulomatous diseases (e.g. tuberculosis, leprosy). Macrophages in granulomas contain 1α-hydroxylase and can produce 1,25-DHCC. The hypercalcaemia is usually readily corrected with glucocorticoids.

What to do if the plasma calcium level is raised

- Consider the clinical history – any evidence of overt or occult malignancy?
- Carefully review the drug history – is the patient taking vitamin D derivatives or calcium supplements?
- Other investigations required may include:
  - PTH, serum phosphate
  - Biochemical/haematology screen may provide clinical clues, e.g. deranged liver function test results
  - Immunoglobulins and serum electrophoresis, Bence Jones protein (exclude myeloma)
  - Tumour workup (chest radiography, faecal occult blood ± colonoscopy, mammography, etc.)
- Institute treatment (see box).

Treatment of hypercalcaemia

Mild hypercalcaemia may not require treatment other than oral hydration and treatment of the underlying cause. Any contributing medications (e.g. calcium supplements, vitamin D, thiazide diuretics) should be stopped. More severe hypercalcaemia increases urinary excretion of sodium and water causing volume depletion and decreased urinary calcium excretion. The first goal of treatment is to replete the extracellular volume with normal saline, which often takes 3–4 L. Loop diuretics will also enhance urinary calcium excretion, but should be used only once the patient has been volume expanded. Adjunctive therapy includes the administration of bisphosphonates, glucocorticoids or calcitonin.

Bisphosphonates impair osteoclastic function and inhibit bone resorption. They are typically given intravenously (e.g. disodium palmidronate 60 mg over 2 h), but if hypercalcaemia is less severe they may be given orally (e.g. alendronic acid 10 mg daily). The hypocalcaemic effect of bisphosphonates typically takes several days. If a more rapid response is required, salmon calcitonin may be used (100–400 units every 6–8 h, subcutaneously). Glucocorticoids (e.g. prednisolone 20–40 mg daily) may be effective for hypercalcaemia associated with granulomatous disorders. Haemodialysis can be considered if other therapies have failed or the serum calcium concentration is markedly raised (4.5–5 mmol/L).

Treatment of hypercalcaemia

- Ensure adequate hydration with intravenous normal saline.
- Intravenous furosemide given to a well hydrated patient promotes urinary calcium loss.
- Bisphosphonates are very effective in malignant disease.
- Steroids may be effective in cases characterised by excess 1,25-DHCC (e.g. sarcoidosis).
- Definitive treatment of the underlying disorder should be planned, e.g. chemotherapy for malignant disease, surgery for severe hyperparathyroidism.
- Other less commonly used treatments include calcitonin, prostaglandin inhibitors (non-steroidal anti-inflammatory drugs), beta-blockers (in thyrotoxicosis), haemodialysis.

Hypocalcaemia

The causes of hypocalcaemia are shown in Table 6.2. Some patients with so-called 'hypocalcaemia' may simply have a reduced plasma protein level, e.g. hypoalbuminaemic patients with severe nephrotic syndrome. Such patients have a normal corrected and ionised calcium level. True hypocalcaemia is commonly due to inadequate levels of active vitamin D. Causes include nutritional deficiency, although this is less common following the addition of vitamin D to foods such as margarine. Malabsorption of vitamin D from the gut may occur in various conditions such as coeliac disease, pancreatic disease or following surgical resection. Renal failure leads to reduced 1,25-DHCC levels as a result of diminished renal 1α-hydroxylase enzyme activity, and liver disease may impair 25-hydroxylation.

Symptoms and complications of hypocalcaemia

- Paraesthesia, e.g. around mouth, fingers
- Muscle cramps
- Increased neuromuscular irritability including tetany – check clinically for Chvostek's sign and Trousseau's sign
- Seizures
- ECG changes – bradycardia, prolonged QT interval
- Calcification of basal ganglia

Table 6.2 Causes of hypocalcaemia

Pseudohypocalcaemia	Secondary to hypoalbuminaemia (normal ionised calcium)
Vitamin D deficiency	See Table 6.3
Decreased PTH action	Autoimmune hypoparathyroidism
	Postparathyroid surgery ('hungry bone' syndrome)
	Hypomagnesaemia
	Pseudohypoparathyroidism (tissue resistance to actions of PTH)
Acute tissue deposition of calcium	Acute pancreatitis
	Rhabdomyolysis
Renal losses	Nephrotic syndrome (loss of vitamin D binding protein)
	Fanconi syndrome
Other	Critical illness/sepsis; multiple blood transfusions (citrate binds calcium and reduces ionised calcium levels)

Rickets and osteomalacia

These conditions may develop in patients with vitamin D deficiency or abnormal vitamin D metabolism (Table 6.3). Adults develop osteomalacia, whereas children develop rickets with its characteristic bony deformities. Patients complain of localised bone pain and tenderness, and may exhibit a proximal myopathy. The biomineralisation of bone is defective and a bone biopsy demonstrates non-mineralised osteoid tissue. Radiography may demonstrate 'pseudo-fractures' or Looser's zones. Disease may also result from genetic deficiency of 1α-hydroxylase or end-organ resistance to the actions of 1,25-DHCC. Clinically similar disease with rickets may result from defective tubular reabsorption of phosphate. In this condition, called hypophosphataemic vitamin D-resistant rickets, there is a low serum phosphate level, marked phosphaturia and no myopathy.

Hypoparathyroidism

This is rare and is characterised by hypocalcaemia, hyperphosphataemia and normal renal function (note that hypocalcaemia and hyperphosphataemia are common in chronic renal failure). The serum PTH concentration is very low or undetectable. Causes include previous parathyroid or thyroid surgery (inadvertent removal of the parathyroid glands), autoimmune disease and infiltrative disorders. The condition

Table 6.3 Causes of vitamin D deficiency

Low vitamin D intake	Low dietary intake (fat-soluble vitamin)
	Low sunlight exposure
Malabsorption	Coeliac disease
	Chronic pancreatitis
	Biliary cirrhosis
	Intestinal bypass, postgastrectomy
Abnormal metabolism	Renal disease (reduced 1α-hydroxylase level)
	Liver disease (reduced 25-hydroxylase level)
	Vitamin D-dependent rickets (25-hydroxylase deficiency)
	Anticonvulsant therapy
Renal losses of vitamin D	Nephrotic syndrome (loss of vitamin D binding protein)
	Fanconi syndrome

of pseudohypoparathyroidism is the result of end-organ insensitivity to the action of PTH, and patients exhibit raised PTH levels.

Miscellaneous conditions

Paget's disease is common in the elderly. Localised areas of the skeleton exhibit increased bone turnover resulting in an increased alkaline phosphatase level, which may be very high. Indeed, Paget's disease is often the cause of an isolated increase in alkaline phosphatase concentration in elderly individuals. Plasma calcium and phosphate levels are usually normal, although patients may become hypercalcaemic during a period of prolonged immobilisation. Osteoporosis is a common bone disorder characterised by a reduced bone mass and an increased fracture risk. Routine biochemical tests show normal calcium and phosphate levels in this condition.

Treatment of hypocalcaemia

Hypocalcaemia is often asymptomatic and can be treated with increased oral calcium intake and supplemental vitamin D. Any underlying cause should be treated. Symptomatic hypocalcaemia (paraesthesia, tetany, seizures, bradyarrhythmias) requires urgent therapy. Intravenous calcium (e.g. 10 mL 10% calcium gluconate over 10 min, followed by slow IV infusion) should be given until the serum calcium level can be maintained by oral calcium and vitamin D supplements. Patients receiving chronic calcium replacement (e.g. in hypoparathyroidism) must be monitored carefully to avoid hypercalciuria, as this can lead to renal stones and nephrocalcinosis.

Caution

Great care must be taken to ensure that intravenous calcium solutions are administered correctly as severe skin necrosis may result if the solution leaks into the tissues.

Phosphate homeostasis

Phosphate is a predominantly intracellular molecule and is found in most foods, but especially dairy produce and animal protein. It plays a key role in cellular energy metabolism (adenosine triphosphate; ATP) and enzyme reactions (e.g. kinases, phosphatases), and is a component of bone (hydroxyapatite). Phosphate levels are controlled by parathyroid hormone (PTH), fibroblast growth factor 23 (FGF23), vitamin D and renal excretion. Normal serum phosphate levels range from to 0.85–1.45 mmol/L.

When should I consider checking a patient's phosphate level?

Consider in patients with:

- renal impairment
- renal tubular disease, e.g. Fanconi's syndrome
- hypoparathyroidism or hyperparathyroidism
- bone disease such as rickets, etc., as this may be secondary to defects in phosphate metabolism
- muscle weakness.

Hyperphosphataemia

Hyperphosphataemia (Table 6.4) is most commonly a problem in kidney disease where decreased glomerular filtration of phosphate occurs. The increased serum phosphate levels may stimulate PTH production by the parathyroid glands (leading to secondary hyperparathyroidism and renal bone disease), or may precipitate with calcium in blood vessels and heart valves. Alternatively, cell lysis with release of intracellular contents may lead to acute hyperphosphataemia; in this condition calcium may be bound, leading to an acute drop in the ionised calcium level and seizures.

Renal bone disease

The commonest cause of hyperphosphataemia is renal impairment. As the glomerular filtration rate falls, the serum phosphate level starts to rise. PTH is stimulated by the rising phosphate concentration, and

Table 6.4 Causes of hyperphosphataemia

Increased absorption	Vitamin D excess
	Phosphate enemas
Cell lysis	Rhabdomyolysis
	Chemotherapy for malignancy
Decreased excretion	Renal impairment
	Hypoparathyroidism

also by low calcium levels and the impaired activation of vitamin D. Renal bone disease is the combination of secondary hyperparathyroidism (increased bone turnover) and low vitamin D levels (osteomalacia). Treatment is aimed at lowering phosphate levels (oral phosphate binders) and replacing activated vitamin D (calcitriol) to lower PTH levels. Note that the raised phosphate levels in combination with high calcium levels (from vitamin D therapy and calcium-containing phosphate binders) may lead to metastatic calcification in blood vessels and cardiac valves. Calcification in small dermal arterioles leads to an ulcerating skin condition called uraemic calcific arteriolopathy, which is often fatal.

Hypophosphataemia

This is often asymptomatic, but in the longer term osteomalacia (in children, rickets) or renal stones secondary to hypercalciuria may develop. At lower levels (serum phosphate <0.4 mmol/L), patients may develop acute symptoms of rhabdomyolysis, muscle weakness (hypoventilation, heart failure) and CNS symptoms (seizure, encephalopathy). See Table 6.5.

Hypophosphataemia in the alcoholic patient

There are multiple reasons for hypophosphataemia in the alcoholic patient who is admitted to hospital. Underlying malnutrition and vitamin D deficiency are compounded by increased urinary phosphate losses from secondary hyperparathyroidism (secondary to vitamin D deficiency) and the toxic effects of alcohol on proximal tubular cells. After admission, a refeeding syndrome may occur, where phosphate is driven into cells by higher insulin levels, glucose phosphorylation and synthesis of new proteins.

Treatment of hypophosphataemia

Acute hypophosphataemia with symptoms requires intravenous phosphate replacement, but this is relatively uncommon. Intravenous phosphate (typically given as potassium phosphate 9 mmol over 12 h) may cause hypocalcaemia or metastatic calcification, and plasma concentrations of calcium and phosphate need to be monitored closely. In most cases, oral phosphate replacement (e.g. Phosphate-Sandoz, 2–6 tablets per day) is sufficient, although diarrhoea is a common side effect.

Table 6.5 Causes of hypophosphataemia

Decreased absorption	Malnutrition
	Phosphate binders (e.g. antacids)
	Chronic diarrhoea
	Vitamin D deficiency (may be secondary to drugs that are P450 enzyme inducers)
Intracellular shift	Glucose phosphorylation (insulin therapy, refeeding syndrome)
	Respiratory alkalosis
Increased urinary losses	Hyperparathyroidism
	Fanconi syndrome
	Oncogenic osteomalacia
	Following kidney transplant
	Hypophosphataemic rickets
	Hereditary hypophosphataemia and hypercalciuria (HHRH)

Magnesium homeostasis

Magnesium is an important and abundant intracellular cation that is involved in many enzymatic reactions. It is contained predominantly within bone and within cells. The plasma magnesium level is closely regulated and, although the exact nature of the homeostatic mechanisms is unclear, regulation of gastrointestinal absorption and renal excretion is important. Unusually for most cations, after glomerular filtration the major site of tubular reabsorption is in the thick ascending limb of the loop of Henle and not the proximal tubule. Although plasma magnesium levels are often poor indicators of total body magnesium reserves, the normal range is 0.7–1.1 mmol/L.

When should I consider checking a patient's magnesium level?

Consider in patients with:

- resistant hypokalaemia
- cardiac arrhythmias
- pregnant women with pre-eclampsia.

Hypomagnesaemia

Hypomagnesaemia is often accompanied by hypokalaemia or hypocalcaemia; the symptoms such as muscular weakness, neurological symptoms (tetany, seizures) and cardiac dysrhythmias are similar. Hypomagnesaemia should be suspected when patients with these conditions fail to respond appropriately to replacement therapy with potassium or calcium. Causes of hypomagnesaemia are listed in Table 6.6. Measurement of urinary magnesium excretion should be performed as this will distinguish between renal and gastrointestinal losses.

Treatment of hypomagnesaemia

Treatment consists of replacement therapy. Oral therapy (e.g. magnesium glycerophosphate) may result in diarrhoea, and in some conditions, such as short bowel syndromes, systemic therapy is required (e.g. intravenous magnesium sulfate).

Hypermagnesaemia

This is an uncommon finding and usually occurs in the context of severe renal failure in a patient taking magnesium supplements (e.g. magnesium-containing laxatives or antacids). Symptoms include gastrointestinal disturbance, muscle weakness (may cause respiratory failure) and bradyarrhythmias (ECG may show a prolonged PR interval, wide QRS and long QT interval).

Table 6.6 Causes of hypomagnesaemia

Increased urinary losses	Diuretics (loop and thiazide diuretics)
	Renal tubular injury (following acute tubular necrosis or kidney transplant)
	Other drugs (aminoglycosides, cisplatin, amphotericin, tacrolimus, alcohol)
	Volume expansion (hyperaldosteronism)
	Gitelman's syndrome
	Familial hypomagnesaemia
Increased gastrointestinal losses	Diarrhoea
	Laxatives

Treatment

Magnesium is a physiological calcium channel blocker, and calcium can reverse this antagonistic action. Intravenous calcium is especially effective for hypotension, dysrhythmias and respiratory distress. Normal saline will expand the extracellular volume and enhance renal elimination.

CHAPTER 7

Liver function tests

Introduction

The term liver function tests (LFTs) refers to a panel of biochemical tests that are often deranged in patients with various forms of liver dysfunction and disease (Table 7.1). The liver may be adversely affected in many diseases, and measuring and monitoring liver function has great clinical utility. It should be recognised that measuring the circulating levels of liver enzymes does not evaluate hepatic synthetic function; this is more appropriately assessed by serum albumin and prothrombin time. The liver performs a number of vital and varied functions including:

- *Synthesis* – the majority of circulating plasma proteins including albumin, coagulation factors and complement components, are synthesised by the liver.
- *Metabolism* – the liver metabolises carbohydrates (gluconeogenesis and the synthesis and breakdown of glycogen), lipids (fatty acid synthesis, cholesterol synthesis, lipoprotein synthesis, ketogenesis), proteins (conversion of amino acids to ammonia [NH_3] and urea) and hormones (25-hydroxylation of vitamin D as well as metabolism of steroid hormones and polypeptide hormones).
- *Excretion* – the liver excretes bile salts and bilirubin, together with many drugs.

Table 7.1 Typical liver function test panel

Test	Normal value (individual labs may vary)
Bilirubin	5–18 μmol/L
Alkaline phosphatase	35–120 iu/L
γ-Glutamyltransferase (GGT)	12–58 iu/L
Aspartate aminotransferase (AST)	5–40 iu/L
Alanine aminotransferase (ALT)	10–60 iu/L
Albumin	35–45 g/L

- *Storage* – the liver stores proteins (allowing complex proteins to be rapidly produced if required), glycogen, fat-soluble vitamins (A, D, K) and vitamin B_{12}.
- *Immunological* – the Kupffer cells within the liver may remove circulating immune complexes, present antigen, etc.

The liver is therefore a key organ and often requires careful biochemical assessment.

Anatomy and physiology

The liver is the largest internal organ in the body and is divided into thousands of functional units called lobules (Fig. 7.1). Each lobule consists of cords of hepatocytes that surround vascular channels called sinusoids. The sinusoids are lined by highly specialised cells of the reticuloendothelial system called Kupffer cells.

The liver receives one-third of its blood supply from the systemic circulation, and the remainder is derived from the portal system. Branches of the hepatic artery and portal vein reach the periphery of a lobule through special tracts called portal triads. Blood percolates to the lobule centre through the sinusoids and drains via a small central vein. Sinusoidal blood is therefore a mixture of arterial and portal blood, and the low PO_2 of sinusoidal blood renders the liver susceptible to hypoxic injury in conditions such as cardiovascular shock.

Hepatocytes produce 1–1.5 L bile per day. Bile is secreted into the biliary canaliculi, which join to form ductules and ultimately the extrahepatic ducts that drain bile to the gallbladder for storage. Bile secreted into the small bowel acts to emulsify lipids into small particles and facilitates the digestive action of the enzyme lipase.

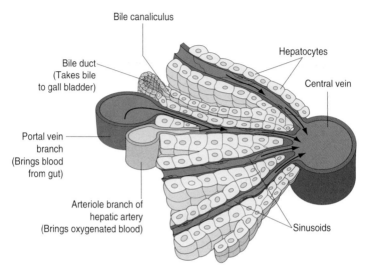

Bile canaliculus

Hepatocytes

Bile duct
(Takes bile
to gall bladder)

Central vein

Portal vein
branch
(Brings blood
from gut)

Arteriole branch of
hepatic artery
(Brings oxygenated blood)

Sinusoids

Figure 7.1 Hepatic lobule.

Thus, bile enhances the breakdown and absorption of fat-soluble nutrients.

Bilirubin metabolism

Bilirubin is a degradation product of haem. Some 80% of haem is derived from haemoglobin and 20% is derived from other haem-containing proteins such as myoglobin and cytochromes. Approximately 300 mg bilirubin is produced per day, although the liver can metabolise and excrete ten times this amount. The excretion of bilirubin can be considered in four steps (Fig. 7.2):

1. *Production of bilirubin* – Haemoglobin released from red cells is bound to haptoglobin in the circulation and this complex is removed by cells of the reticuloendothelial system located principally in the spleen. The haem ring is cleaved to produce the tetra-pyrrole bilirubin and this unconjugated (hydrophobic) form circulates in the plasma bound to albumin.
2. *Conjugation and secretion of bilirubin* – In the liver the bilirubin is detached from albumin by hepatocytes and transported to the

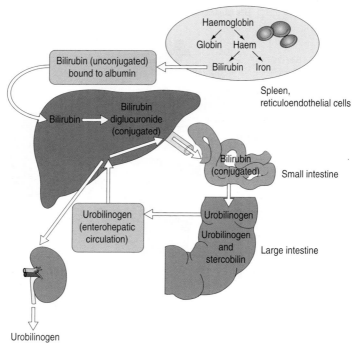

Figure 7.2 Bilirubin excretion and the enterohepatic circulation.

smooth endoplasmic reticulum. The bilirubin is then conjugated with glucuronic acid to form water-soluble conjugated bilirubin (bilirubin diglucuronide), which is secreted into the biliary canaliculi for excretion in the bile.

3. *Intestinal metabolism of bilirubin* – Bilirubin is degraded by bacteria within the colon and urobilinogen is generated. This is then converted to urobilin or the pigmented stercobilin, which imparts a dark brown colour to faeces.

4. *Enterohepatic circulation* – Some of the water-soluble urobilinogen is reabsorbed from the colon into the portal blood and returned to the liver for biliary excretion. However, small amounts of water-soluble urobilinogen do reach the systemic circulation and are excreted in the urine.

Direct and indirect bilirubin

In normal individuals 95% of circulating bilirubin is unconjugated and bound to albumin. The systemic circulation contains only very small amounts of conjugated bilirubin as a result of minor leakage from hepatocytes. Conjugated bilirubin is described as 'direct reacting' because of its water solubility. Unconjugated or 'indirect' bilirubin must be solubilised in alcohol or other agents before being assayed in common tests. The total and direct bilirubin is typically measured and the difference between the two values used to calculate the level of indirect bilirubin.

Bile salts

Bile salts comprise 70–90% of bile and are synthesised by hepatocytes from cholesterol conjugated to glycine or taurine. The commonest bile salts are cholic acid and chenodeoxycholic acid. They act to solubilise cholesterol and prevent gallstone formation, and emulsify fats in the intestine in order to facilitate the digestion and reabsorption of fat. Bile salts are normally reabsorbed in the colon by the enterohepatic circulation and recycled to the liver. Bile salts are a sensitive indicator of structural liver disease but are not measured routinely. Bile salts accumulate in blood in biliary obstruction and are responsible for the intense itching complained of by patients.

Alkaline phosphatase (ALP)

This enzyme is predominantly found in liver (biliary tract and liver epithelial cells) and bone (osteoblasts), but may also be found in granulocytes, intestinal epithelial cells and renal proximal tubular cells. Circulating ALP is derived predominantly from liver, bone and intestine (10–20%) and has a half-life of approximately 7 days. Therefore, raised ALP levels may also be found in non-hepatic conditions such as bone disease (Paget's disease, bony metastases), late pregnancy (placental ALP) and some intestinal disorders. ALP levels may be raised 2–3-fold in rapidly growing adolescents, and may be increased slightly (1.5-fold) in older adults. In obstructive liver disease, damage to biliary duct epithelial cells results in the release of ALP, which then leaks into the circulation.

γ-Glutamyltransferase (GGT)

This enzyme is found predominantly in hepatocytes and biliary epithelium, but also at lower levels in kidney, pancreas, liver, spleen, heart, brain and seminal vesicles. It may increase in biliary obstruction but may also be induced by alcohol and drugs such as phenytoin.

Aminotransferases

Alanine aminotransferase (ALT) is a cytoplasmic enzyme that is relatively liver specific. ALT has a half-life of 37–57 h and the level tends to become raised at an early stage in hepatic injury.

Aspartate aminotransferase (AST) is a cytoplasmic and mitochondrial enzyme in hepatocytes, but is less liver specific as it is also found in cardiac muscle, skeletal muscle kidney and brain tissue. It has a shorter half-life (12–22 h), but levels may be raised to a greater degree in chronic conditions.

When should I consider checking a patient's liver function?

LFTs are now performed routinely in many patients, but there are still a number of specific indications including:

- jaundice
- suspected neoplasm (?metastases)
- excess ethanol ingestion
- suicidal overdoses (?paracetamol)
- sepsis and very ill patients (?shock liver)
- acute abdominal pain (?gallstones)
- viral illnesses
- diabetes (fatty infiltration)
- a coagulation disorder.

The detection of minor abnormalities in liver function is a common finding with the widespread use of multi-channel analysers. Abnormal LFT results can be broadly classified according to the pattern of enzyme abnormalities into:

- an isolated abnormality, such as an increased level of bilirubin or ALP alone
- obstructive LFT findings, characterised predominantly by a rise in ALP and GGT levels
- hepatocellular injury, characterised predominantly by a rise in AST and ALT levels.

Increased serum bilirubin concentration may occur in conditions resulting in an obstructive pattern of LFTs as well as in hepatocellular injury, and is thus less specific. Indeed, a clear distinction between cholestatic disease and hepatocellular injury is not always possible as they may coexist. For example, acute hepatitis often has a marked cholestatic element at later stages.

In most patients with abnormal LFT results a diagnosis can be obtained non-invasively. A liver biopsy may be required in patients with an unclear diagnosis, and the commonest findings include alcoholic liver disease, steatosis or steatohepatitis.

What do I do with the result?

For the sake of simplicity, this will be broken down into sections depending upon the primary pattern of the LFT result, categorised as:

- Jaundice pattern with significant increase in bilirubin concentration alone
- Obstructive pattern with raised ALP and GGT levels
- Hepatocellular pattern with increased ALT and AST levels.

Jaundice (with increased levels of bilirubin alone)

> Mild jaundice will pass unnoticed as jaundice is clinically detectable only when the serum bilirubin level is greater than 50 µmol/L.

See Figure 7.3 for a breakdown of the causes of jaundice.

Haemolysis

Increased release of haemoglobin from cells undergoing haemolysis generates large amounts of bilirubin. If liver function is normal, the rise in serum bilirubin concentration will be largely unconjugated (bound to serum albumin) as the liver is able to excrete large amounts of conjugated bilirubin. The increased amounts of conjugated bilirubin in the gut produce increased urobilinogen, which may be absorbed via the enterohepatic circulation and increase urinary urobilinogen levels. Haemolysis may be detected by the combined measurement of haemoglobin, the reticulocyte count and haptoglobin levels, coupled with scrutiny of the blood film. The level of serum bilirubin is rarely greater than 70 µmol/L in haemolytic conditions.

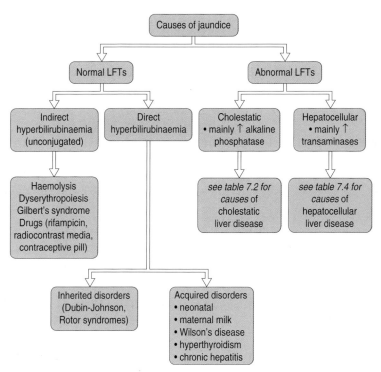

Figure 7.3 Causes of jaundice.

Gilbert's syndrome

This is a common inherited condition occurring in approximately 5% of the population, more commonly in males. Bilirubin is conjugated with glucuronic acid by UDP–glucuronosyltransferase, a family of enzymes derived from multiple splice variants of a single gene. A common polymorphism in the promoter sequence of this gene impairs the rate of transcription. Individuals with impaired enzyme levels or function have a persistent mild unconjugated hyperbilirubinaemia (<80 µmol/L) with otherwise normal LFTs. Patients are clinically unaffected, although they may become noticeably jaundiced at times of illness or fasting.

Obstructive pattern of LFTs with raised ALP and GGT levels

The conjugation of bilirubin may be normal in this setting, but the excretion of bile into the gut is hindered. Conjugated bilirubin levels rise in the plasma, and the water-soluble conjugated bilirubin may be found in the urine imparting a dark yellow colour. The absence of urobilinogen and hence stercobilinogen in the gut results in pale coloured faeces.

Levels of ALP and GGT are typically raised in hepatic and biliary obstruction. To confirm whether the ALP is of hepatic origin it is possible to measure tissue specific isoenzymes, but this is rarely performed because the associated increase in GGT concentration is sufficient corroborative evidence of a hepatic source for the ALP. It should be noted that low ALP values may be seen in hypothyroidism, pernicious anaemia, zinc deficiency, congenital hypophosphataemia and fulminant Wilson's disease complicated by haemolysis. Raised levels of GGT are less specific than ALP, as increased levels may be found in pancreatic disease, myocardial infarction, renal failure and chronic obstructive pulmonary disease. An isolated increase in GGT concentration with otherwise normal LFT findings should not lead to exhaustive testing for liver disease (see below).

Learning points

- Bilirubin in the urine suggests hepatobiliary disease as it is only water-soluble conjugated bilirubin that can be excreted in the urine.
- Cholestasis is suggested by raised alkaline phosphatase (ALP) and γ-glutamyltransferase (GGT) levels.
- Cholestasis may be present in the absence of jaundice.
- The combination of ALP and GGT measurement provides a sensitive marker of liver metastases that rivals radiological imaging.
- A low serum albumin level suggests a chronic process owing to its long half-life (~20 days), whereas a normal albumin concentration implies an acute process (e.g. acute hepatitis, gallstones).

There are many causes of obstructive LFTs that may be divided into causes of extrahepatic and intrahepatic cholestasis (Table 7.2).

Table 7.2 Causes of cholestatic liver disease

Extrahepatic cholestasis

- Cholelithiasis
- Malignancy (carcinoma of head of the pancreas or ampulla, cholangiocarcinoma), portal lymphadenopathy
- Primary sclerosing cholangitis
- Miscellaneous – AIDS cholangiopathy (cytomegalovirus [CMV], cryptosporidium, human immunodeficiency virus [HIV]), chronic pancreatitis, biliary stricture, parasitic infection (ascariasis, liver fluke).

Intrahepatic cholestasis

- Alcoholic hepatitis
- Primary biliary cirrhosis
- Non-alcoholic steatohepatitis
- Drugs – myriad! (Table 7.3)
- Secondary to hepatocellular injury, e.g. viral hepatitis and secondary tissue oedema
- Sepsis
- Infiltrative disease – amyloid, lymphoma, sarcoid, tuberculosis
- Miscellaneous conditions – total parenteral nutrition, cholestasis of pregnancy, postoperative cholestasis, vanishing bile duct syndrome, various rare syndromes (Dubin–Johnson, Rotor), paraneoplastic syndrome (Stauffer's syndrome), Caroli's disease, thyrotoxicosis, protoporphyria.

Table 7.3 Drugs and liver disease

Predominantly hepatocellular injury

Paracetamol, salicylates, tetracyclines, azathioprine, methotrexate, ferrous sulphate, antituberculous agents (isoniazid, rifampicin), amiodarone, halothane, methyldopa, dantrolene, anticonvulsants (sodium valproate, phenytoin), NSAIDs, ketoconazole, beta-blockers, tacrine, propylthiouracil

Predominantly cholestatic injury

Androgens, phenothiazines (chlorpromazine, haloperidol), hypoglycaemic agents (chlorpropamide, tolbutamide), antibiotics (nitrofurantoin, erythromycin, co-trimoxazole, penicillins), phenytoin, imipramine, sulindac, cimetidine, oestrogens, immunosuppressive agents (ciclosporin, azathioprine), hydralazine, captopril, carbimazole

Alcohol and GGT

The synthesis of GGT is induced by alcohol as well as drugs such as phenytoin, barbiturates and rifampicin. Levels take 3–6 weeks to return to normal following cessation of alcohol intake, and levels of this enzyme are used to monitor patients in alcohol abuse programmes.

Patterns of enzyme rises

In liver disease, levels of ALP and GGT are usually increased together in roughly equal amounts. Variations to this pattern may provide clues to particular diagnoses:

- *Raised ALP with normal GGT levels* – this suggests a non-hepatic cause of the increased ALP concentration, e.g. bone disease, intestinal disease, pregnancy, adolescence.
- *Isolated increase in GGT level* – this suggests excess alcohol consumption or other liver enzyme inducers, e.g. rifampicin, phenytoin and barbiturates. A raised GGT level may also be found in pancreatic disease, myocardial infarction and renal failure.

The degree of increase of these markers may also provide diagnostic clues:

- A marked increase in ALP concentration (up to 10–20 times normal) is suggestive of primary biliary cirrhosis or extrahepatic biliary obstruction with malignant obstruction, typically causing higher bilirubin levels than obstruction secondary to gallstones.
- A marked increase in both ALP and GGT levels with a disproportionate rise in GGT concentration suggests drug-induced cholestasis, with resultant induction of GGT synthesis.
- Hepatocellular injury may not affect solely ALT and AST, but may also increase ALP and GGT levels 2–3-fold.
- Fluctuating levels may suggest the presence of intermittent obstruction, as may occur in patients with gallstones.
  See Figure 7.4 for initial investigation of cholestatic LFTs.

Learning points

- Raised levels of aminotransferases (AST and ALT) suggest hepatocellular injury.
- The degree of increase in the concentration of aminotransferases does not correlate with the degree hepatocellular injury on biopsy, but may be used to follow the course of disease.

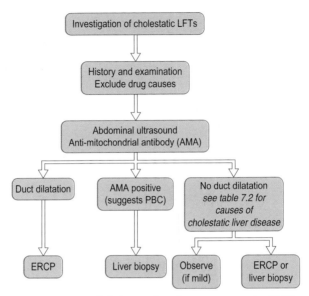

Figure 7.4 Investigation of cholestatic liver function test results. ERCP, endoscopic retrograde cholangiopancreatography.

Hepatocellular pattern with increased ALT and AST levels

The liver has a large functional reserve and minor injury may not be reflected by changes in LFT results. Moderate injury may result in raised levels of transaminases, with cholestatic changes and jaundice appearing as the hepatocellular injury worsens. Abnormalities in the synthetic function of the liver are evident in cases of marked hepatocellular injury.

Patterns of raised aminotransferase levels

The degree of increase in the levels of aminotransferases may provide diagnostic clues:

1. *Marked increase* (up to 20 times normal) – this suggests conditions such as acute viral hepatitis, shock liver (ischaemic hepatitis) or acute drug/toxin hepatotoxicity such as paracetamol poisoning. Less common causes include acute Budd–Chiari syndrome, veno-occlusive disease, the HELLP syndrome (*h*aemolytic anaemia, *e*levated *l*iver enzymes and *l*ow *p*latelet count) or acute fatty liver of

pregnancy, hepatic infarction and acute exacerbation of autoimmune chronic active hepatitis. It is important to note that a sudden fall in AST and ALT levels in the absence of clinical improvement is an ominous sign as it implies exhaustion of viable hepatocytes.

2. *Moderately raised levels* (3–10 times normal) – this may be seen with infectious mononucleosis, chronic hepatitis, extrahepatic obstruction, Reye's syndrome, myocardial infarction, etc.

3. *Mildly raised levels* (1–3 times normal) – may be found in pancreatitis, alcoholic fatty liver, granulomatous/neoplastic hepatic infiltration, primary biliary cirrhosis, etc.

Note

Normal aminotransferase levels are often found in patients with chronic hepatitis C infection.

The AST : ALT ratio

Usually the AST and ALT levels are raised to a similar degree, with a ratio of approximately 0.8 (see Figure 7.5 for investigation). In some conditions the AST concentration is increased to a greater degree, resulting in a high ratio. This may occur in:

1. Alcoholic hepatitis – a ratio >2 is suggestive of alcoholic hepatitis but it may be as high as 5. Note that the sources of AST may be partly extrahepatic, e.g. seizures and rhabdomyolysis that result in release of AST from muscle tissue.
2. Hepatitis C with cirrhosis.
3. Non-alcoholic steatohepatitis.
4. Liver metastases – the AST rise may be marked compared with the ALT rise.
5. Non-hepatic disease, e.g. muscle disorders, myocardial infarction, thyroid disorders, coeliac disease, false-positive increase in AST concentration with erythromycin treatment.

By contrast, a low AST : ALT ratio may be seen with:

1. Acute inflammation – ALT is a more sensitive and early marker of hepatocellular injury, e.g. post-transfusion hepatitis, occupational toxic exposure.
2. Cholestasis – extrahepatic obstruction is an acute process resulting in a greater rise in ALT concentration. The reverse may be present with intrahepatic obstruction.

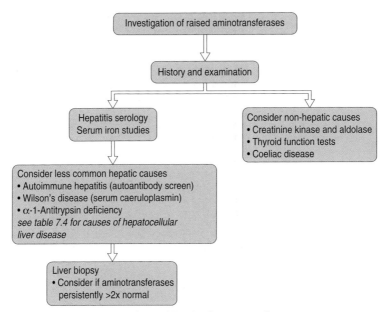

Figure 7.5 Investigation of raised levels of aminotransferases.

Postoperative jaundice

This is a common finding and is typically multifactorial with aetiological factors including (Table 7.4):

- increased erythrocyte breakdown (haematoma, transfusion of stored blood)
- possible hepatocellular damage resulting from drugs, anaesthetic agents, hypotensive shock, etc.
- intrahepatic cholestasis, e.g. sepsis, hypotension, total parenteral nutrition
- surgical injury to bile ducts should also be considered.

Assessment of hepatic synthetic function

The serum albumin and prothrombin time are used to assess hepatic synthetic function and the severity of the liver injury. Very severe liver

Table 7.4 Causes of hepatocellular injury

Group of causes	Specific
Viral	Hepatitis viruses (HAV, HBV, HCV), herpes viruses, haemorrhagic viruses (yellow fever, Ebola, Marburg, Lassa), adenoviruses, enteroviruses
Drugs	See Table 7.3
Alcohol and toxins	Chlorinated hydrocarbons (carbon tetrachloride; chloroform), amanita phylloides (mushroom poisoning), aflatoxin B1, arsenic, phosphorus
Immunological	Autoimmune hepatitis, non-alcoholic steatohepatitis
Specific liver conditions	Wilson's disease, haemochromatosis, α1-antitrypsin deficiency, porphyrias, liver infiltration (amyloid, lymphoma, sarcoid)
Neoplasms	Metastatic liver disease, hepatocellular carcinoma, lymphoma
Vascular	Congestive heart failure, shock liver, tricuspid incompetence, constrictive pericarditis, Budd–Chiari syndrome, veno-occlusive disease
Other infections	*Bacterial* – tuberculosis, leptospirosis, syphilis, pyogenic abscess, brucella, rickettsia
	Fungal – candida, blastomyces, coccidioides, histoplasma, cryptococcus
	Parasitic – helminths (ascaris, fasciola, clonorchis, schistosomiasis, echinococcus), protozoa (amoebiasis, plasmodia, babesiosis, toxoplasmosis, leishmaniasis)

injury may be associated with a low serum urea concentration as a result of failure of urea production together with hypoglycaemia.

Albumin

The liver synthesises 12–15 g albumin each day. The serum half-life of albumin is 17–20 days and it therefore takes about 3 weeks of liver injury before the serum albumin levels fall. Pre-albumin (transthyretin) has a half-life of 2 days and offers a more accurate assessment of hepatic synthetic function in patients with acute liver injury. It is important to be aware that hypoalbuminaemia is non-specific and may also be seen in patients with malnutrition, protein-losing enteropathy or nephrotic syndrome.

Coagulation factors

The liver is responsible for the production of many coagulation factors. Four of these factors (prothrombin and factors VII, IX and X) are dependent on vitamin K for that post-translational modification of the proteins that is required for their functional activity.

The coagulopathy associated with liver disease may be due to:

1. hepatocellular dysfunction
2. vitamin K deficiency, as cholestasis results in impaired absorption of fat-soluble vitamins including vitamin K.

Vitamin K treatment will thus help to distinguish between these possibilities and will almost always rapidly correct the coagulation abnormality secondary to extrahepatic jaundice (<12 h). It should be noted that cholestasis may occur in association with hepatocellular dysfunction and treatment with vitamin K may be partly effective in this setting.

Factor VII has the shortest half-life of the coagulation factors. As a result, the prothrombin time (PT) becomes prolonged at an early stage, and PT is the most sensitive measure of coagulation in liver dysfunction. PT >5 s above normal should raise concern of a fulminant course in acute viral or toxic hepatitis. PT >100s is an indication for liver transplantation.

Patients with chronic liver disease exhibit prolongation of both the PT (factors II, VII, X) and the activated partial thromboplastin time (factors II, IX, X). The levels of fibrinogen and factor V fall at a late stage in severe liver failure and abnormalities of other factors are usually responsible for the coagulation defects.

In clinical practice, coagulation abnormalities due to hepatocellular injury may not require correction as the raised PT is often not clinically serious and may be a useful parameter to monitor disease severity. The PT is one of the parameters employed in the Child–Pugh classification of the severity of liver disease (Table 7.5). Treatment with vitamin K and fresh frozen plasma should be considered when there is active bleeding (usually gastrointestinal) or before invasive procedures.

Urea and ammonia

The nitrogenous products of protein metabolism are converted in the liver to ammonia and then to urea in the urea cycle. In severe liver disease this pathway breaks down and serum levels of urea may fall. Some 90% of liver function must be lost before urea production is impaired. Ammonia is generated in the gut by bacteria and is a potent

Table 7.5 Child–Pugh classification of severity of liver disease. The patient is scored from 1 to 3 for each of the five categories

	Points assigned		
	1	2	3
Bilirubin (μmol/L)	<28	28–51	>51
Albumin (g/L)	>35	28–35	<28
Prothrombin time (seconds > control)	1–3	4–6	>6
Ascites	Absent	Slight	Moderate
Encephalopathy	None	Grade 1–2	Grade 3–4
Child–Pugh grade	A (well compensated)	B (significant functional compromise)	C (decompensated)
Score	5–6	7–9	10–15
1-year survival (%)	100	80	45
2-year survival (%)	85	60	35

neurotoxin. In liver disease, the serum levels of ammonia may rise due to inadequate hepatic conversion to urea. This may also be due to shunting of portal blood away from hepatocytes. Raised ammonia levels have been associated with hepatic encephalopathy in severe liver disease.

Glucose

During fasting, the liver plays an important role in maintaining blood sugar levels by glycogenolysis (breakdown of stored glycogen) or gluconeogenesis (generation of glucose from amino acids or free fatty acids). This protective mechanism may be impaired in severe liver dysfunction, such as during fulminant acute liver necrosis, thereby resulting in hypoglycaemia. Patients may require regular monitoring of blood sugar levels.

Clinical assessment

The underlying cause of the abnormal LFT results, as well as the severity of liver dysfunction, may be suggested by the pattern of the abnormalities (Table 7.6) and by taking a full history and performing a thorough physical examination. Specific features to look for include the following.

Clinical history

- Presence of jaundice, change in stool or urine colour, itch (obstructive jaundice)
- Abdominal pain, fever, rigors, jaundice (gallstones, ascending cholangitis)
- Arthralgias, myalgia, anorexia, rash (drugs, hepatitis)
- Alcohol consumption
- Exposure to drugs, medications and herbal remedies
- Disorientation, memory loss (encephalopathy)
- Easy bruising, bleeding, black stools (coagulopathy, bleeding oesophageal or gastric varices)
- Previous history of injections, blood transfusions, intravenous drug use and tattoos together with sexual history (risk factors for hepatitis)
- Occupational history, e.g. exposure to industrial toxins, farming (hydatid disease), sewage workers (leptospirosis), healthcare workers (hepatitis)

Table 7.6 Patterns of abnormal liver function tests

	Gilbert's/ haemolysis	Acute hepatitis	Chronic hepatitis	Cirrhosis	Cholestasis	Malignancy
Bilirubin	↑	N or ↑↑	N or ↑	N or ↑	↑ or ↑↑↑	N
ALP	N	N or ↑	N	N or ↑↑	↑↑↑	↑↑
GGT	N	N or ↑	N	N or ↑↑	↑↑↑	↑↑
Aminotransferases	N	↑↑↑	↑	N or ↑	N or ↑	N or ↑
Albumin	N	N	N or ↓	N or ↓	N	N or ↓
Immunoglobulins[a]	N	N	↑	↑	N	N
Prothrombin time	N	N or ↑	N or ↑	N or ↑	N or ↑[b]	N

N, normal.
[a]IgA levels increased in cirrhosis; IgG levels increased in autoimmune hepatitis.
[b]May correct with vitamin K.

- Other – travel history, contaminated food, history of previous gall-stones, abdominal surgery, family history of liver disease.

Examination

- Degree of jaundice
- Clinical stigmata of chronic liver disease
- General (spider naevi, hepatomegaly, parotid enlargement, muscle wasting)
- Hands (finger clubbing, leuconychia, Dupuytren's contracture)
- Disturbed endocrine function (gynaecomastia, impotence, decreased body hair, testicular atrophy, palmar erythema)
- Portal hypertension (splenomegaly, ascites, peripheral oedema, caput medusa, rectal varices)
- Liver failure (hepatic fetor, encephalopathy, flapping tremor)
- Cardiovascular system – raised jugular venous pressure (congestive cardiac failure with hepatic congestion, tricuspid incompetence, constrictive pericarditis)
- Presence of lymphadenopathy (neoplasm, lymphoma), Kayser–Fleischer ring (Wilson's disease), hyperpigmentation (haemochromatosis, primary biliary cirrhosis) or xanthomata (primary biliary cirrhosis).

Special tests

Hepatitis serology in liver disease

Acute hepatitis is usually secondary to hepatitis viruses (A–E) (Table 7.7), but other systemic viral infections (Epstein–Barr virus, CMV, HIV) or toxins (alcohol, paracetamol, carbon tetrachloride, fungal toxins) may produce a similar clinical picture. Transaminase levels may be greatly increased.

Initial screening hepatitis serology consists of testing for hepatitis B surface antigen (HBsAg) and antihepatitis C antibody. A higher index of suspicion or positivity on initial screening tests prompts further testing.

Hepatitis A (HAV)

This infection is spread by the faeco-oral route and is more common in children and those living in poor sanitary conditions. Clinically, an incubation period of 2–6 weeks is followed by malaise, nausea and anorexia. An icteric illness follows that rarely lasts longer than 6 weeks. Fulminant hepatitis occurs in less than 0.3% of cases. Chronic

Table 7.7 Clinical features of hepatitis viruses

	Hepatitis A	Hepatitis B	Hepatitis C	Hepatitis D	Hepatitis E
Route of infection	Faeco-oral	Parenteral	Parenteral	Parenteral	Faeco-oral
Incubation period	2–6 weeks	2–6 months	2–52 weeks	3–13 weeks	3–6 weeks
Onset	Abrupt	Insidious	Insidious	Abrupt	Abrupt
Chronic carriage	No	Yes	Yes	–	No
Acute mortality rate	<0.3%	1–4%	<1%	30%	1–2% (pregnant women 20%)
Progression to end-stage liver disease	No	Rare	25%	–	No

hepatitis or progression to cirrhosis does not occur. The diagnosis is confirmed by the presence of IgM anti-HAV antibodies or increasing titres of IgG anti-HAV antibodies.

Hepatitis B infection

This virus is acquired parenterally, most commonly by transfusion, needle-sharing or sex. After a 2–6-month incubation period, an acute illness develops in about 50% of infected adults, with fulminant hepatitis occurring in about 1% of cases. Patients may develop chronic hepatitis or an asymptomatic chronic carrier state (HBsAg positive, but HBV e antigen [HBeAg] and HBV DNA negative). Levels of transaminases are typically normal in the carrier state. HBV infection is assessed by measuring HBsAg, HBV core antigen (HBcAg) and HbeAg, together with their corresponding antibodies (Table 7.8).

Hepatitis C infection

This virus is acquired parenterally, often through intravenous drug use or therapeutic blood products. The acute infection is usually mild and subclinical. However, only 10–15% of infected individuals eradicate

Table 7.8 Serological markers of hepatitis B infection

Marker	Time of appearance after infection	Clinical implication
HBsAg	4–12 weeks	Earliest indicator of acute infection. Persistence >6 months indicates chronic infection
HBeAg	4–12 weeks	Indicates viral replication and associated with high infectivity
HBcAg	–	Not detectable in serum
Anti-HBs antibody	4–10 months	Indicates previous infection and immunity to further HBV infection
Anti-HBe antibody	8–16 weeks	Indicates resolution of acute infection
Anti-HBc IgM antibody	6–14 weeks	Indicates acute infection with HBsAg
HBV DNA	4–12 weeks	Used to assess viral replication and suitability for antiviral treatment

the virus and chronic infection is the typical course. Over 10–20 years, cirrhosis and later hepatocellular carcinoma commonly develop. The presence of HCV antibody demonstrates exposure to the virus (appears 12–16 weeks after infection), and viraemia (HCV RNA) may be detected by the polymerase chain reaction (PCR).

Autoantibody screen in liver disease

A polyclonal increase in immunoglobulin levels is common in many types of liver disease, particularly raised IgA levels (detected by performing plasma protein immunoelectrophoresis and measuring serum immunoglobulins). IgG levels are markedly increased in chronic hepatitis, and IgM levels are raised in primary biliary cirrhosis. Specific autoantibodies may be associated with a number of hepatic diseases.

Autoimmune hepatitis

This condition occurs more commonly in young women and has a variable presentation ranging from chronic abnormalities on LFTs to severe acute hepatitis and cirrhosis. Extrahepatic manifestations may be prominent, including haemolytic anaemia, thrombocytopenia, thyroiditis, colitis and type 1 diabetes mellitus. Antinuclear antibodies (ANAs) are positive in autoimmune hepatitis, although non-specific, with anti-double-stranded DNA antibodies typically being absent. More specific autoantibodies include anti-smooth muscle antibodies (SMAs) and anti-liver and kidney microsomal antibodies. It should be noted that approximately 5% of patients with chronic hepatitis C infection have a positive ANA result, and anti-SMA and anti-liver and kidney microsomal antibodies have also been described.

Primary biliary cirrhosis (PBC)

A positive anti-mitochondrial antibody is highly specific for PBC, with the disease typically presenting as cholestatic liver disease. PBC predominantly affects women; clinical features include itch, hyperpigmentation and hepatomegaly. PBC may also be associated with other autoimmune diseases.

Other circulating antibodies such as antineutrophil cytoplasmic antibodies (ANCAs) may be found in chronic liver diseases such as primary sclerosing cholangitis and autoimmune hepatitis.

α1-Antitrypsin (α1-AT)

This glycoprotein is an antiprotease that inhibits the action of several proteases, including trypsin and plasmin, and thereby acts to prevent excessive tissue destruction and scarring. Allelic variants of the gene are common and may result in low serum α1-AT concentrations. Affected individuals are predisposed to the development of early-onset emphysema and liver injury with cirrhosis. The variant α1-AT accumulates in hepatocytes and is detectable on liver biopsy. The condition is suggested by the absence of the α1 peak on plasma protein electrophoresis and is confirmed by measuring serum α1-AT levels and determining the α1-AT phenotype.

Serum caeruloplasmin

Low levels of the copper transport protein caeruloplasmin (<20 mg/dL) are suggestive of Wilson's disease. This is an autosomal recessive condition resulting from mutations in the P-type ATPase that inhibits the cellular export of copper. This results in the intracellular accumulation of copper in certain tissues, particularly liver and brain. Clinically patients often present at a young age with liver disease secondary to hepatocellular injury or cirrhosis, or with neuropsychiatric disorders. Corneal deposits of copper may produce the characteristic Kayser–Fleischer rings on slit-lamp examination. Confirmatory investigations include a high 24-h urinary copper excretion (usually >100 µg/d, normal <30 µg/d) and evidence of copper accumulation on liver biopsy. Note that about 10% of patients with Wilson's disease have normal serum caeruloplasmin levels.

Serum iron studies

Raised serum iron levels are suggestive of haemochromatosis. This is a common autosomal dominant condition resulting from mutations in the *HFE* gene and causing increased iron absorption from the gastrointestinal tract and subsequent iron overload. The iron is deposited in tissues, particularly liver, heart and pancreas. Clinical features include liver disease (hepatomegaly, abnormal LFT results, cirrhosis, hepatocellular carcinoma), diabetes mellitus, skin pigmentation ('bronze diabetes'), arthropathy and cardiomyopathy. The diagnosis of haemochromatosis is supported by iron studies revealing an increased transferrin saturation (>45%) and a raised serum ferritin level (>400 ng/mL in men and >300 ng/mL in women). The definitive investigation is a liver biopsy that demonstrates parenchymal iron deposition by Prussian blue staining. In some centres genetic testing for the common C282Y and H63D mutations may be available.

α-Fetoprotein (AFP)

Levels of this serum tumour marker are raised in patients with hepatocellular carcinoma and may be measured in those at risk of developing this tumour, e.g. patients with established cirrhosis. The level of AFP correlates with tumour size and may reach levels >10 000 ng/mL (normal <30 ng/mL) in patients with large undifferentiated tumours. However, it should be noted that a mild increase in AFP (~500 ng/mL) may be found in patients with cirrhosis or hepatitis in the absence of malignant disease. In addition, AFP levels may also be increased in some testicular tumours and AFP is used as a maternal marker for fetal neural tube defects.

Other tumour markers

The level of carcinoembryonic antigen (CEA) may be measured in patients with cholestatic abnormalities on liver function testing. It is usually normal in those with benign biliary strictures, but may be raised (~3-fold) in patients with primary sclerosing cholangitis or cholangiocarcinoma (~5-fold). CA19-9 concentration may be increased in ductal pancreatic carcinoma.

CHAPTER 8

Lipid disorders

Introduction

The two main lipids in the blood are cholesterol and triglycerides. They are hydrophobic and circulate in plasma bound to apoproteins in complexes known as lipoproteins. Cholesterol is essential for the formation of cell membranes, steroid hormone production and bile acid formation. Triglycerides are important in energy utilisation.

Hypercholesterolaemia is a major risk factor for coronary artery disease. Cholesterol lowering in patients with known cardiovascular disease (secondary prevention) leads to a decreased mortality across population groups. The data in patients without known cardiovascular disease (primary prevention) is less clear, but in those at high risk (patients with diabetes or multiple risk factors) lipid lowering is recommended.

Classification of lipoproteins

Lipoproteins consist of a core of hydrophobic lipid (triglyceride and cholesterol esters) surrounded by hydrophilic phospholipids and non-esterified cholesterol. Apolipoproteins are found on the surface and play key roles in regulating lipoprotein metabolism.

Lipoproteins are classified into five major types depending on their density (Table 8.1).

Exogenous (dietary) pathway

Cholesterol and fatty acids are absorbed from the small bowel. Within the cells of the intestinal mucosa, fatty acids combine with glycerol to

Table 8.1 Classification of lipoproteins

	Size[b] (nm)	Percentage lipid concentration[a]		Major apolipoprotein
		Triglyceride	Cholesterol	
Chylomicron	>200	80–95%	2–7%	B-48
VLDL	30–140	55–80%	5–15%	B-100
IDL	23–27	20–50%	20–40%	B-100
LDL	19–22	5–10%	40–50%	B-100
HDL	7–13	5–10%	15–25%	A-I

[a]Remaining percentage consists of apolipoprotein. VLDL, very low density lipoprotein; IDL, intermediate density lipoprotein; LDL, low density lipoprotein; HDL, high density lipoprotein.
[b]Size is variable, and small dense LDL particles may be more atherogenic.

form triglycerides, and cholesterol is esterified. These lipids are bundled with apolipoproteins to form chylomicrons, which enter the circulation (Fig. 8.1).

Lipoprotein lipase in the capillaries of peripheral tissues hydrolyses core triglycerides, releasing free fatty acids to be used as an energy source or stored in adipose tissue. The end-product of metabolism is the chylomicron remnant, which is taken up by the liver.

Endogenous pathway

This pathway conveys lipids from the liver to peripheral tissues or in the reverse direction (reverse cholesterol transport) (Figs. 8.2 & 8.3).

Very low density lipoprotein (VLDL) is synthesised by the liver and enters the circulation. VLDL is hydrolysed by lipoprotein lipase (in the capillaries of fat and muscle tissue), depleting triglyceride and leading to the generation of intermediate density lipoprotein (IDL). The IDL is either cleared from circulation by the low density lipoprotein (LDL) receptor or remodelled by hepatic lipase to form LDL. LDL may be taken up by the liver (LDL receptor), where it is converted to bile acids and secreted into intestinal lumen, or may be transported to non-hepatic tissues, incorporated into cell membranes, steroid hormone production or stored as cholesterol esters. Defects in the LDL receptor lead to familial hypercholesterolaemia.

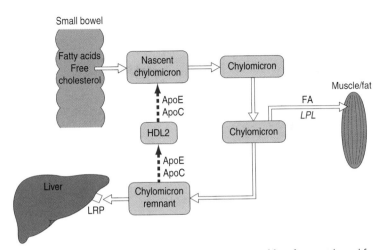

Figure 8.1 Exogenous (dietary) pathway. Absorption of free fatty acids and free cholesterol from the small bowel with delivery of fatty acids (FA) to peripheral tissues and uptake of the chylomicron remnants by the liver. Apo, apolipoprotein; LPL, lipoprotein lipase; LRP, LDL receptor-related protein.

De novo cholesterol synthesis

This occurs within cells via hydroxymethylglutaryl-coenzyme A (HMG-CoA) reductase. Statins decrease the activity of this enzyme, resulting in a fall in intracellular cholesterol levels, increasing LDL receptor expression, and thus lowering serum LDL levels.

Reverse cholesterol transport

High density lipoprotein (HDL) is formed in the liver and in intestinal cells from phospholipid and apolipoproteins, and procures further surface components (apolipoproteins, cholesterol and phospholipid) from chylomicron remnants and IDL (Fig. 8.3).

HDL can remove free cholesterol from intracellular sources, such as atherogenic foam cells, (reverse cholesterol transport), accounting for its antiatherogenic effect. Other effects may be maintenance of endothelial function and of low blood viscosity via red cell deformity.

There is an inverse relationship between plasma HDL cholesterol levels and cardiovascular risk. HDL levels lower than 1 mmol/L

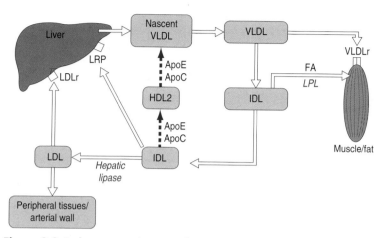

Figure 8.2 Endogenous pathway. Trafficking of lipids from the liver to peripheral tissues and the production of LDL. VLDL is produced by hepatocytes and released into the circulation where it matures and undergoes lipolysis of the triglyceride component by lipoprotein lipase (LPL) in capillaries perfusing muscle and fat to form IDL. Further lipolysis by hepatic lipase leads to the formation of LDL, which is removed by the liver via the LDL receptor (LDLr) or may be taken up by peripheral tissues, promoting atherosclerosis and tissue injury. FA, fatty acids.

increase the risk of coronary artery disease (CAD) by about 20%. In contrast, HDL levels greater than 1.9 mmol/L are associated with a longer lifespan.

Hyperlipidaemia and atherosclerosis

Atherosclerotic plaques in the arterial walls of patients contain large amounts of cholesterol. Circulating LDL that is not taken up by LDL receptors may be taken up by macrophages via scavenger receptors (CD36). Accumulation of excess cholesterol in these cells produces foam cells, which contribute to the atherosclerotic plaque. Oxidised LDL is more atherogenic and is taken up preferentially by macrophages.

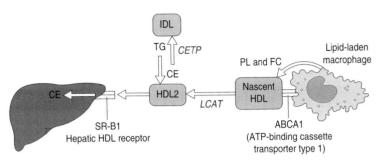

Figure 8.3 HDL metabolism: reverse cholesterol transport. This mechanism transports surplus lipids from peripheral tissues (including atherogenic foam cells) back to the liver. Promotion of this pathway by new therapeutic agents could potentially reduce atherosclerosis. ABCA1, ATP-binding cassette transporter type 1; CE, cholesterol ester; CETP, cholesterol ester transfer protein; FC, free cholesterol; LCAT, lecithin cholesterol acyltransferase; PL, phospholipid; SR-B1, scavenger receptor class B type 1; TG, triglycerides.

Measurement of the lipid panel

> The level of LDL cholesterol ('bad cholesterol') correlates with the risk of coronary artery disease, whereas HDL cholesterol ('good cholesterol') is protective against coronary artery disease.

Who should be checked?
- Any patient with cardiovascular disease (coronary artery disease, stroke, peripheral vascular disease)
- All patients with diabetes mellitus
- Other patients at high risk for hyperlipidaemia (thyroid disease, liver disease, renal disease)
- Cardiovascular risk assessment – it is recommended that all individuals over 40 years old should undergo a cardiovascular risk assessment.

How should a lipid panel be measured?
- 12-h fast (meal or acute alcohol can increase the triglyceride level).

- Wait for 3 months postmyocardial infarction (but can be measured accurately within the first 24 h after myocardial infarction).
- Note that the LDL concentration is a calculated level and may be inaccurate when the triglyceride (TG) level is >5 mmol/L.
- Measurement of the ratio of total cholesterol to HDL is often used to assess the significance of a raised total cholesterol (TC). As HDL is protective, a low ratio is beneficial.
- If the cholesterol level is raised, the patient should be assessed further for secondary causes (diabetes, renal disease, proteinuria, liver disease, alcohol intake, hypothyroidism).

Non-HDL cholesterol

In patients with raised TG levels (>5 mmol/L), calculated LDL levels are inaccurate, and some use non-HDL cholesterol levels (TC − HDL). The target for non-HDL cholesterol in individuals at high risk for cardiovascular disease is <3 mmol/L.

Hypercholesterolaemia

Data from large epidemiological studies have shown that about 50% of the adult industrialised population have a total cholesterol level >5 mmol/L and about 20% have a TC level >6 mmol/L.

Note: Total cholesterol levels do not differentiate between the amounts of cholesterol carried by LDL and HDL. Women often have higher HDL levels, and for a given TC level may be at lower risk for CAD. It is therefore important to consider the whole lipid panel and not merely the total cholesterol.

Example:

Patient A: TC 7.1, LDL 3.5, HDL 2.8, TG 1.7 mmol/L
Patient B: TC 7.1, LDL 5.4, HDL 0.6, TG 2.3 mmol/L

Although TC is the same for both patients (7.1 mmol/L), patient B has a much higher risk of CAD because the LDL level is markedly increased and the HDL level is low (high TC:HDL cholesterol ratio).

Familial hypercholesterolaemia

Patients with markedly raised LDL levels (>5 mmol/L) often have genetic forms of hypercholesterolaemia and require early detection and family screening (Table 8.2). Familial hypercholesterolaemia occurs in 5–10% of individuals who develop CAD before the age of 55 years.

LDL receptor mutations

This common condition is due to mutations in the gene encoding the LDL receptor. Homozygous patients are rare, but have extremely high levels of LDL (8-fold greater than normal) and present with atherosclerotic disease in childhood. Heterozygotes have LDL concentrations twice normal (total cholesterol usually >9 mmol/L) and develop premature CAD in their thirties and forties. Patients may have tendon xanthomas, tuberous xanthomas or xanthelasma. A similar phenotype may be caused by mutations in apolipoprotein (Apo) B-100.

LCAT deficiency

Lecithin cholesterol acyltransferase is important in reverse cholesterol transport. Deficiency is an autosomal recessive disease with corneal clouding, target cell haemolytic anaemia and proteinuric renal failure. The lipid panel shows increased TC and TG levels, with a decreased HDL concentration.

Combined hypercholesterolaemia and hypertriglyceridaemia

Familial combined hyperlipidaemia

This is the most common form of dyslipidaemia, accounting for 1 in 300 of the adult population. It appears to be autosomal dominant, although expression is variable.

Dysbetalipoproteinaemia

ApoE mediates the uptake of lipoproteins by the LDL receptor and the LDL receptor-associated protein (LRP). There are three major ApoE

Table 8.2 Causes of hypercholesterolaemia

Primary lipid disorders	Type II familial hypercholesterolaemia
	Type I, IV, V hyperlipoproteinaemia
Secondary causes	Cholestasis/liver disease, nephrotic syndrome/ proteinuria, hypothyroidism, pregnancy, drugs (progestogen, ciclosporin, thiazides)

alleles (E2, E3, E4). ApoE2 has a lower affinity for the LDL receptor, and homozygotes for this variant may have severe hyperlipidaemia. Tuberous xanthomas and striae palmaris (cholesterol deposits in palmar creases) may be present. Note that 1% of the population is homozygous for ApoE2, mostly with normal lipid levels, so a second factor is required.

Hypercholesterolaemia in certain conditions

Diabetes mellitus

Hyperlipidaemia is usually not a prominent feature of type 1 diabetes as long as blood sugar control is adequate. In type 2 diabetes, the typical pattern is of hypertriglyceridaemia with low HDL levels. This lipid pattern is partly due to the associated obesity and insulin resistance. The term 'metabolic syndrome' has been applied to the constellation of features of central obesity, dyslipidaemia, hypertension, gout and type 2 diabetes. Patients with diabetes are at a greatly increased risk of CAD, and the target levels for TC and LDL cholesterol are the same as for those with established CAD (LDL <2 mmol/L).

Renal disease

Chronic kidney disease and haemodialysis are typically associated with hypertriglyceridaemia and low HDL cholesterol. Proteinuria and nephrotic syndrome may be associated with profound hypercholesterolaemia secondary to increased lipoprotein production by the liver. Renal transplant patients commonly have hypercholesterolaemia, as least partly secondary to the immunosuppressive medications (calcineurin inhibitors, steroids). Note that patients undergoing haemodialysis, despite being at very high cardiovascular risk, tend to have low levels of LDL.

Liver disease

Cholestatic liver disease typically causes hypercholesterolaemia. By contrast, acute liver injury may be associated with low cholesterol levels.

Cardiovascular risk assessment

Guidelines for cardiovascular risk assessment and treatment have been published recently by the Joint British Societies (Heart 2005; 91 (Suppl 5):V1–V52).

When considering lipid-lowering therapy a comprehensive cardiovascular risk assessment should be performed (Table 8.3). It is recommended that all individuals over the age of 40 years undergo cardiovascular disease risk assessment in primary care. All patients with diabetes aged over 40 years are considered to be at high risk.

A patient's 10-year risk of developing cardiovascular disease can be estimated using the Joint British Societies' cardiovascular risk prediction charts. Copies of these charts may be found at the back of the British National Formulary (BNF). If concomitant hypertriglyceridaemia (>1.7 mmol/L) is present, the risk should be multiplied by 1.3.

Clinical management of hypercholesterolaemia

Lipid targets in high-risk patients (Joint British Societies [JBS2])

Total cholesterol (TC) <4 mmol/L and
LDL cholesterol (LDL) <2 mmol/L
  or
25% reduction in TC level and 30% reduction in LDL concentration[a]

[a]whichever is lower.

Table 8.3 Risk factors for cardiovascular disease

Non-modifiable risk factors	Modifiable risk factors
Age	Smoking
Male sex	Dyslipidaemia
Family history of cardiovascular disease	(hypercholesterolaemia, low HDL, hypertriglyceridaemia)
	Hypertension
	Diabetes mellitus
	Kidney disease and albuminuria
	Obesity
	Physical inactivity
	Stress

The treatment of hypercholesterolaemia should not be considered in isolation, but rather in the context of overall management of cardiovascular risk (Fig. 8.4). Other measures include smoking cessation, blood pressure control and blood sugar control. Exercise and weight loss should also be implemented. Aspirin should be given if the cardiovascular risk is high enough to consider intervention.

Diet

Dietary therapy typically lowers LDL cholesterol by only 5–10%, although some patients have a more marked response, and it is often appropriate to begin therapy with a low cholesterol diet. A weight loss strategy is also important in many patients. In patients with a marked increase in LDL cholesterol or established cardiovascular disease, drug therapy is likely to be required to achieve targets.

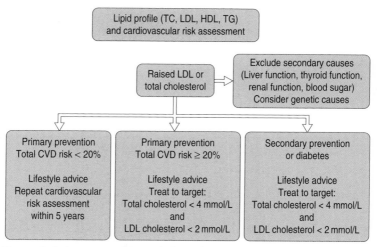

Figure 8.4 Assessment of hypercholesterolaemia. Cardiovascular risk is assessed by the Joint British Societies' cardiovascular disease risk chart (Heart 2005; 91(Suppl 5):V1–V52).

Lipid-lowering (statin) treatment?

Treatment decisions should be based upon the patient's LDL cholesterol level and their cardiovascular risk assessment (including HDL level). In general, lowering LDL cholesterol by 1 mmol/L reduces the risk of cardiovascular disease by 25–30%.

It is recommended that lipid-lowering (statin) treatment (and other cardiovascular disease protective therapies) be given to:

1. All patients with established cardiovascular disease (secondary prevention)
2. Patients with diabetes mellitus (type 1 or type 2)
   – All those aged >40 years
   – Those with an additional risk factor (retinopathy, nephropathy or microalbuminuria, HbA1c >9%, hypertension, TC >6 mmol/L, positive family history of premature CVD, metabolic syndrome)
3. Individuals with total CVD risk >20% over 10 years
4. Individuals with a TC : HDL cholesterol ratio ≥6.0.

Target of lipid-lowering therapy in high risk patients

The goal of lipid-lowering therapy is to reduce TC levels to <4 mmol/L and LDL cholesterol to <2 mmol/L. In those with hypertrigyceridaemia, in whom LDL levels cannot be calculated, the goal is a non-HDL cholesterol level of <3 mmol/L.

> **Importantly, patients at highest risk for coronary artery disease or those with established disease may be started on statin therapy irrespective of the cholesterol level.**

Hypertriglyceridaemia

Triglyceride accounts for 95% of stored fat, but circulates predominantly as VLDL (80%) and LDL (15%). Patients with marked hypertriglyceridaemia are at risk for pancreatitis. Recent studies also suggest that raised TG levels are an independent risk factor for cardiovascular disease.

Causes of hypertriglyceridaemia

See Table 8.4.

Table 8.4 Causes of hypertriglyceridaemia

Primary lipid abnormalities (genetic disorders)	Hyperlipoproteinaemia (I, IIb, III, IV, V) (familial combined hyperlipidaemia, familial hypertriglyceridaemia, familial dysbetalipoproteinaemia)
Secondary causes	Metabolic syndrome, alcoholism, type 2 diabetes, chronic kidney disease, pregnancy, stress/sepsis, drugs (oestrogen, beta-blockers, thiazides, steroids, sirolimus, protease inhibitors)

Lipoprotein lipase deficiency

Mutations in the gene encoding lipoprotein lipase (LPL), the enzyme that enables peripheral tissues to take up TG from chylomicrons and VLDL, lead to massive accumulation of chylomicrons. These patients have marked hypertriglyceridaemia and present with recurrent pancreatitis, lipaemia retinalis, eruptive xanthomas and hepatosplenomegaly at a young age. ApoC-II deficiency is a rare autosomal recessive disorder that causes a functional LPL deficiency.

Metabolic syndrome

Increased TG levels are an important feature of the metabolic syndrome, found in a subgroup of patients with a greatly increased risk of coronary heart disease. Features of this syndrome include central obesity, dyslipidaemia (TG >1.7 mmol/L, HDL <1 mmol/L [men] or <1.3 mmol/L [women]), hypertension (blood pressure >130/85 mmHg) and glucose intolerance.

Clinical management of hypertriglyceridaemia

Individuals with a TG level >1.7 mmol/L should be investigated for secondary causes. The primary therapy for hypertriglyceridaemia is dietary. Additional measures include weight loss, exercise, avoiding alcohol, improving blood sugar control in patients with diabetes, and increasing omega-3 fatty acid intake by increasing fish consumption (Fig. 8.5).

In patients with TG levels >6 mmol/L, the immediate risk is of acute pancreatitis and urgent therapy is required. In other patients with lesser degrees of hypertriglyceridaemia, the primary concern is of

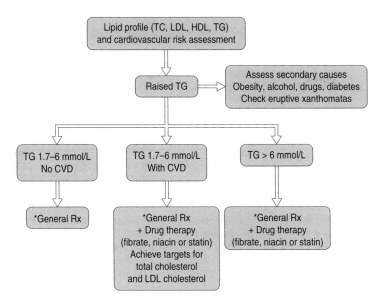

Figure 8.5 Management of hypertriglyceridaemia. *General Rx = diet, exercise, weight loss, reduce alcohol, control diabetes, increase omega-3 fatty acid intake through fish consumption. CVD, cardiovascular disease.

cardiovascular risk, and drug therapy (using fibrates, niacin or statins) should be considered in those with other risk factors.

Lipid-lowering drugs

HMG-CoA reductase inhibitors (statins)

These agents inhibit the rate-limiting step in the endogenous pathway of cholesterol synthesis and lead to an increased cellular expression of LDL receptors, removing increased amounts of cholesterol from the circulation (Table 8.5). They typically reduce LDL cholesterol by 30–40%. Examples of these medications include atorvastatin, simvastatin and pravastatin.

Adverse effects include myositis and abnormal liver function test results, and these should be assessed before starting these agents and if the patient subsequently develops symptoms. The risk of

Table 8.5 Effect of drug therapy on lipoprotein levels

	LDL	HDL	TG
Statins	−25 to −40%	+5 to −10%	↓ to ↓↓
Fibrates	−10 to −15%	+15 to 20%	↓↓
Niacin	−15 to −25%	+25 to 35%	↓↓
Cholestyramine	−15 to −25%	–	–
Ezetimibe	−15 to −20%	–	–

myositis may be higher in patients concurrently taking fibrates or niacin, or in transplant patients taking calcineurin inhibitors.

Fibrate derivatives

These drugs raise HDL cholesterol and lower TG levels. They are typically used for combined hypertriglyceridaemia and hypercholesterolaemia. Examples include gemfibrozil and fenofibrate. Adverse effects of fibrates include cholelithiasis, hepatitis and myositis.

Bile acid binding resins

These agents (cholestyramine, colestipol) act by binding bile acids in the gut and interrupting the enterohepatic circulation. This causes the liver to increase bile acid production, using more cholesterol. These agents decrease LDL levels by 15–25% with no effect on HDL, and may increase the TG concentration. They should not be used in patients with significant hypertriglyceridaemia.

The use of bile acid binding resins may be complicated by gastrointestinal symptoms (constipation, flatulence), and they may interfere with the absorption of drugs or fat-soluble vitamins.

Ezetimibe

This is a new lipid-lowering agent that blocks the intestinal absorption of cholesterol. It reduces LDL levels by 15–20% as monotherapy, but can enhance LDL reduction on those already taking a statin.

Nicotinic acid

This drug raises HDL cholesterol and lowers TG levels. Intolerance is common and only about 50% of patients can tolerate a full dose. The main complaint is prostaglandin-mediated flushing or pruritus. Other side effects include exacerbation of gout, peptic ulcer disease and glucose intolerance.

Omega-3 fatty acids
These may be used to lower TG levels and prevent coronary heart disease.

Hypocholesterolaemia

Some patients may present with abnormally low levels of total cholesterol (<2.6 mmol/L). This usually reflects malnutrition or underlying chronic disease (Table 8.6). Occasionally, rare primary disorders of lipid metabolism may produce this phenotype.

Table 8.6 Causes of hypocholesterolaemia

Primary lipid abnormalities	Hypo-α-lipoproteinaemia, hypo-β-lipoproteinaemia, Tangier disease, lecithin cholesterol acyltransferase (LCAT) deficiency
Secondary causes	Severe liver disease, malnutrion/malabsorption, hyperthyroidism, acute illness, myeloproliferative disorders, chronic anaemia

CHAPTER 9

Markers of cardiac and muscle injury and disease

The measurement of a variety of intracellular enzymes and structural proteins in plasma can indicate the presence of severe cellular damage or necrosis. Such tests are particularly useful in patients with suspected cardiac or muscle disease. For example, the ischaemic necrosis of cardiac myocytes occurring during myocardial infarction (MI) results in the release of intracellular proteins and enzymes into the circulation. As a result, detection of these usually sequestered molecules provides information regarding both the presence and the extent of muscle damage.

Creatine kinase (CK) consists of dimers of M and B chains, and therefore there are three potential isoenzymes (MM, MB and BB). CK is a cytosolic enzyme that facilitates the mitochondrial transfer of high-energy phosphates from the cytoplasm. It is widely distributed in tissues but is found predominantly in muscle. Skeletal muscle contains approximately 99% CK-MM and about 1% CK-MB. However, during muscle fibre regeneration following skeletal muscle injury, the amount of CK-MB may increase. Cardiac myocytes contain 20–30% CK-MB, with the remainder being CK-MM. The CK-BB isoform is found in other organs such as the brain, and is not routinely measured. Under normal circumstances, CK-MM accounts for more than 95% of circulating CK.

Creatine kinase levels

Although individual laboratory assays vary, the normal level of total CK is ~55–170 U/L (males) and ~30–135 U/L (females), although individuals with large muscles may have higher levels. The relative specificity of the CK-MB isoform for myocardial tissue has proved useful in the investigation of patients with suspected cardiac disease. In order to confirm a diagnosis of acute MI, a 2-fold increase is typically required with an increase in the CK-MB fraction (normal CK-MB level 0–5 ng/mL; acute MI >9 ng/mL). Alternative measurements include determining the ratio of CK-MB to total CK, with a ratio >2.5 suggesting a cardiac source.

CK levels usually increase by 4–6 h following a MI, peak at 18–24 h and fall to normal by 36–48 h (Fig. 9.1 & Table 9.1). Serial testing of cardiac enzymes is usually performed to ensure that raised levels are not

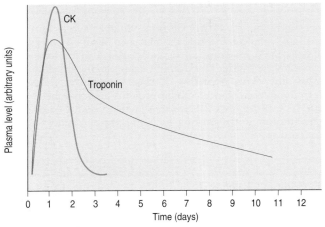

Figure 9.1 Time course of cardiac enzymes/proteins following myocardial infarction. CK, creatine kinase.

Table 9.1 Markers of myocardial infarction

Test	Onset	Peak	Duration
CK (total and MB)	3–12 h	18–24 h	36–48 h
Troponins	3–12 h	18–24 h	Up to 10 days
LDH	6–12 h	24–48 h	6–8 days
Myoglobin	1–4 h	6–7 h	24 h

missed and to guide prognosis. Most cases of acute MI will demonstrate raised levels of CK by 12 h. However, it should be noted that this marker is not as sensitive as cardiac troponins (see below), and a 'small MI' with limited myocardial injury (a 'microinfarct') may not be detected using measurement of CK alone. CK levels are not raised during an episode of angina or pericarditis. It is important to note that an increased CK-MB level may occur in muscle injury with regenerating fibres (e.g. marathon runners, extensive rhabdomyolysis or myositis). However, in these settings the typical acute rise and fall in CK-MB levels is absent.

A cardiac cause for a raised CK level is suggested by:

- Clinical history of chest pain, etc.
- Typical time course (rapid rise within 4–6 h and fall to normal by 36–48 h)
- Raised CK-MB level (>9 ng/mL)
- Increased ratio of CK-MB : total CK (>2.5).

An acute MI should not be diagnosed on a single blood sample for cardiac markers. The rise and fall of levels in the appropriate timescale is also required.

Clinical use of creatine kinase in cardiac disease

1. Diagnosis of acute MI.
2. Assessment of prognosis following acute MI, as the total quantity of CK released (the area under the curve) correlates with infarct size.
3. Assessment of coronary artery reperfusion. The peak level of CK reflects the kinetics of washout from the injured myocardium and is less strongly correlated with infarct size. Thus, successful reperfusion following an angioplasty or thrombolysis leads to an increased

early peak level of CK-MB with a shorter duration due to 'washout' of the enzyme from the affected region of myocardium.

4. Diagnosis of an additional MI or extension of the original infarct. The short duration of raised CK-MB levels (36–48 h) does not permit the late diagnosis of an acute MI if the patient presents several days after chest pain. However, it does mean that CK-MB levels can be used to detect an additional MI or extension of the original infarct. These events may not be detected using troponin levels, which remain increased for a prolonged period after MI.

Non-cardiac causes of raised CK levels

- Skeletal muscle injury – myopathies, myositis, muscular dystrophies, muscle injury, surgery, convulsions, intramuscular injections
- Brain injury (stroke)
- Hypothyroidism

Cardiac troponins

Troponins are structural proteins present within cardiac myocytes. They are involved in the interaction between the contractile proteins actin and myosin, although there is also a cytosolic pool. The two main troponins are cardiac troponin I (cTnI) and cardiac troponin T (cTnT). A MI is associated with an early rise in troponins due to release from the cytoplasmic pool, and a later sustained rise secondary to breakdown of structural actin and myosin filaments. Troponins are not released during purely ischaemic episodes with no cardiac muscle damage.

Troponin I is specific to cardiac myocytes, whereas troponin T is expressed to a minor degree in skeletal muscle. However, both troponins are considered relatively specific for myocardial injury. Cardiac troponin levels begin to rise 4–6 h post-MI with a time course similar to that of CK-MB, but a blood sample taken 12 h after the clinical event is required to detect increases in all patients (also true for CK-MB). The levels of cardiac troponins remain raised for up to 10 days after a MI. This is useful as it facilitates a diagnosis of MI to be made when patients present to hospital or their GP several days after an episode of severe chest pain when the CK-MB levels are normal, as they return to baseline by 36–48 h. However, subsequent rises in CK-MB may permit the diagnosis of infarct extension or an additional MI.

Cardiac troponin levels

Cardiac troponins are normally not detected in blood. The normal level for cTnT is <0.01 μg/mL, and any significant increase represents myocardial injury. The European Society of Cardiology/American College of Cardiology cutoff for acute MI is 0.03 μg/mL. In general, the levels of cardiac troponins reflect infarct size and correlate with prognosis.

There are multiple assays for cTnI that recognise different complexes of serum troponin I, and local reference ranges should be sought for this measurement. In general, levels >1.5 ng/mL suggest significant myocardial injury.

Note:

- Although cardiac troponins are specific for myocardial injury, increased levels may occur in acute pulmonary embolism (due to acute right ventricular strain) and myocarditis (CK-MB levels are often normal in myocarditis).
- A false-positive increase in cardiac troponin levels may occur in chronic renal failure (CRF). Some 10–15% of patients with CRF exhibit mildly raised levels of troponin T and 5% have increased levels of troponin I. The aetiology is unclear.
- Heparin in plasma samples can bind cTnT, reducing levels by 15–30%. Therefore, troponins should be measured in serum samples.

Clinical use of cardiac troponin levels

1. *Diagnosis of acute MI.* Raised levels are sensitive markers of myocardial injury and are especially useful in settings where CK-MB levels may be increased from non-cardiac tissue, e.g. in patients with concurrent skeletal muscle injury or following surgery.
2. *Prognosis of acute MI.* The extent of increase correlates with infarct size and subsequent patient prognosis.
3. *Late diagnosis of acute MI.* The level of cardiac troponins remains increased for up to 10 days after MI, thereby permitting a late diagnosis.
4. *Exclusion of acute MI in patients with chest pain.* Cardiac troponins are very sensitive markers of myocardial injury and normal levels at 12 h post chest pain may be used to exclude MI. This is especially

important in the assessment of patients presenting to the emergency department with chest pain.

5. *Diagnosis of 'microinfarction'*. Troponins are more sensitive than CK-MB, and the term microinfarction has been applied to low-level increases in troponin levels with negative CK-MB levels. These patients would previously have been classified as having unstable angina, but the group with raised cardiac troponin levels has been shown to have a worse prognosis.

When should I check cardiac enzymes and troponin levels?

These should be checked in:

- Patients with an acute coronary syndrome, e.g. unstable angina, MI with ECG changes
- Patients with a history suggestive of prolonged myocardial ischaemia but in whom the diagnosis of an acute coronary syndrome is unclear
- Following surgical coronary revascularisation or percutaneous interventions
- Consider in patients who become suddenly unwell, e.g. develop hypotension or dyspnoea. Remember that elderly patients, especially diabetic individuals, may have a 'silent' MI without any chest pain and that MI may complicate other conditions such as sepsis or surgery.

Assessment of acute MI

Any patient presenting with chest pain requires:

- a thorough history and examination
- electrocardiography
- cardiac markers (troponins and CK-MB) to assess myocardial injury – therapy should not be withheld pending these levels.

Definition of acute MI

An acute MI is diagnosed by the combination of a typical rise and fall of markers of myocardial necrosis (troponins or CK-MB) in association with one of the following:

1. Symptoms of myocardial ischaemia
2. Development of pathological Q waves on ECG
3. ECG changes typical of myocardial ischaemia (ST segment elevation or depression)
4. Coronary artery intervention (e.g. angioplasty).

Previously CK (particularly the CK-MB fraction) was used, but the more specific cardiac troponins have become the 'gold standard'.

Note:

- No single marker can successfully identify or exclude acute MI within the first 6 h.
- A negative cardiac troponin test at 12 h excludes an acute MI in a patient presenting with chest pain.

Other markers of myocardial injury

Lactate dehydrogenase (LDH)

LDH has five different isoenzymes (LDH1–5). Although LDH5 predominates in skeletal muscle (and liver), and LDH1 and LDH2 predominate in the heart, analysis of isoenzymes is rarely performed in clinical practice. LDH is a non-specific marker of tissue injury as its concentration is raised in myocardial injury, malignancy, liver disease, lung disease, kidney disease and haemolysis. Indeed, LDH levels are monitored serially in patients with ongoing haemolysis, e.g. haemolytic uraemic syndrome. LDH levels remain increased for 5 days post-MI and were previously useful in the diagnosis of acute MI after CK levels had returned to normal. This has been superseded by the measurement of cardiac troponins.

Aspartate aminotransferase (AST) and myoglobin

AST is also non-specific and its concentration is raised in skeletal muscle disease, haemolysis and liver disease. Myoglobin is a small protein that is rapidly released from damaged tissue, and could potentially be used as an early marker of acute MI. However, it is not measured routinely as it is non-specific for cardiac muscle and is raised in all forms of muscle injury.

Additional tests in acute myocardial infarction

Haematological tests

Acute MI is often associated with a leucocytosis (typically 12–$15 \times 10^3/mm^3$) and a raised erythrocyte sedimentation rate (ESR) and C-reactive protein (CRP) level, which begins by day 2–3 and can last for several weeks. In patients who develop a prolonged increase of the ESR and CRP level associated with chest discomfort, a diagnosis of Dressler's syndrome is suggested.

Lipid panel

The levels of total cholesterol and high density lipoprotein (HDL) remain close to baseline for 24–48 h, but then rapidly fall. In view of the important role of lipid-lowering agents in secondary prevention, a lipid panel should be checked within the first 48 h or after 8 weeks when the levels are once again close to baseline.

Disorders of skeletal muscle

Patients with a wide range of disorders may present with muscle weakness or myalgia, and require careful investigation. The muscle enzymes measured in clinical practice include creatine kinase (CK), lactate dehydrogenase (LDH), alanine aminotransferase (ALT), aspartate aminotransferase (AST) and aldolase.

Creatine kinase

This is present in the highest concentrations in the serum and is the most sensitive marker of muscle injury (see above). Normal skeletal muscle contains approximately 99% of the CK-MM isoform, but injured muscle undergoing regeneration, as in inflammatory myopathies or after extreme exertion, may have an increased content of the CK-MB isoform and this can occasionally lead to confusion with myocardial injury. However, measurement of cardiac troponin levels will resolve this issue.

Creatine kinase levels in muscle disorders

Normal serum CK levels are less than 170 U/L but can be markedly increased in muscle injury or disease (Table 9.2). Very high levels may be seen with rhabdomyolysis, acute myositis (polymyositis, dermatomyositis, etc.) and Duchenne muscular dystrophy early in the course of the disease (CK levels fall later as muscle loss ensues).

Rhabdomyolysis

This refers to acute muscle necrosis and may be seen in trauma/crush injuries, compartment syndromes and muscle ischaemia, or following fits or electrocution, but any severe acute muscle injury may cause this syndrome. Rhabdomyolysis may result in acute renal failure secondary

Table 9.2 CK levels in muscle disorders

Creatine kinase level	Muscle disorder
Markedly increased (CK > 10 000 U/L)	Rhabdomyolysis
	Myositis: polymyositis, dermatomyositis
	Muscular dystrophy, e.g. Duchenne muscular dystrophy, Becker muscular dystrophy
	Malignant hyperthermia
Moderately increased (CK 1000–10 000 U/L)	Muscle injury/surgery
	Acute myositis (inclusion body myositis, infection, cocaine abuse, adverse effect of statin)
	Other muscular dystrophies
Mildly increased (CK <500–1000 U/L)	Myotonic dystrophy
	Female carriers of Duchenne muscular dystrophy
	Congenital myopathies
	Hypothyroid myopathy
	Intramuscular injections (for 48 h)
Normal levels	Myasthenia gravis
	Thyrotoxic myopathy
	Steroid myopathy
	Neurogenic causes of muscular atrophy, e.g. poliomyelitis, motor neurone disease

to myoglobin-mediated tubular toxicity, although an additional insult such as hypotension or sepsis may also be required. There is anecdotal evidence for the beneficial effect of urinary alkalinisation by the administration of sodium bicarbonate in patients with renal impairment. Typically, very high serum CK levels (>15 000 U/L) are found. In addition, patients often exhibit:

- Marked hyperkalaemia and hyperphosphataemia – potassium and phosphate are released from the damaged muscle.
- Hypocalcaemia – it is thought that the calcium precipitates in damaged muscle. No treatment is required and 25% of patients develop mild hypercalcaemia in the recovery phase.
- An increase in creatinine concentration that is out of proportion to the urea, as creatinine is derived from muscle.

Other muscle enzymes

Lactate dehydrogenase

This enzyme catalyses the last step of glycolysis, the conversion of lactic acid to pyruvic acid. LDH is present in nearly every tissue and, although it is a marker of cell necrosis, the lack of specificity limits its diagnostic utility.

Aminotransferases

These enzymes catalyse the conversion of alanine (alanine aminotransferase, ALT) and aspartate (aspartate aminotransferase, AST) to α-ketoglutarate, providing a source of nitrogen for the urea cycle. Their levels may be raised in a wide number of conditions, especially hepatic, skeletal muscle and myocardial diseases as well as haemolysis (aminotransferases are discussed further in Chapter 7).

Aldolase

This is a glycolytic pathway enzyme found in all tissues, but predominantly in skeletal muscle, liver and brain. Aldolase levels are often raised in muscle disorders, and rarely may be increased in myositis when CK levels are normal.

Special tests associated with muscle disease

When muscle disorders are suspected from increased muscle enzyme levels, further testing may be useful.

Autoimmune screen

This may help to identify autoimmune disease associated with muscle disease, e.g. systemic lupus erythematosus (SLE), polymyositis, dermatomyositis or rheumatoid arthritis. General screening tests should include antinuclear antibody and rheumatoid factor. If polymyositis or dermatomyositis is considered, further testing for antibodies such as anti-Jo-1, anti-nRNP, anti-Scl-70, anti-Sm, anti-La and anti-ENA should be considered.

Anti-acetylcholine receptor antibody

This autoantibody is present in approximately 80% of patients with myasthenia gravis and is virtually diagnostic of the disease. Note, however, that 20% of patients with myasthenia gravis will have a negative result.

Thyroid function tests

Both hypothyroidism and hyperthyroidism may be associated with muscle disease and should be excluded. *Note:* Other endocrine disorders may also present with muscle weakness, e.g. adrenal insufficiency, diabetes, acromegaly.

Serum electrolytes (calcium, potassium and phosphate)

Muscle weakness may be associated with hypercalcaemia and, in particular, with hyperparathyroidism. Vitamin D deficiency leads to osteomalacia and a proximal myopathy. An acute myopathy, even rhabdomyolysis, may result from either hypokalaemia or hypophosphataemia.

Genetic testing

Genetic tests are available for some of the congenital myopathies and dystrophies, such as Duchenne muscular dystrophy; this may permit more accurate genetic counselling.

CHAPTER 10

Immunological investigations

Introduction

Immunological disease is not uncommon (Box 10.1) and is responsible for considerable morbidity and mortality. The immune system comprises the innate and adaptive immune system and has evolved to protect the host from various pathogens including bacteria, viruses, protozoa, fungi, helminths, etc. The innate immune system comprises neutrophils, monocytes, macrophages, complement, etc. Although the innate immune system may combat infection, it is complemented by the more highly evolved adaptive immune system. This comprises dendritic cells that process pathogen-derived antigens and present them to T cells in association with major histocompatibility complex (MHC) class II molecules. This initiates the immune response characterised by clonal T-cell proliferation and activation, as well as the maturation of B cells into antibody-producing plasma cells. Importantly, the adaptive immune system is characterised by 'immunological memory' such that a robust immune response can be generated more effectively following repeat exposure to the same pathogen, a feature exploited in vaccination programmes (Fig. 10.1).

A key requirement of an effective immune system is the ability to discern 'self antigens' from 'non-self antigens', as would be found on pathogens. Autoimmune disease is the result of a breakdown in this tolerance (Fig. 10.2), although the underlying mechanisms remain

Box 10.1 Autoimmune conditions characterised by autoantibody generation

- Various connective tissue disorders including:
  - systemic lupus erythematosus (SLE)
  - rheumatoid arthritis
  - scleroderma
  - dermatomyositis
  - Sjögren's syndrome
- ANCA-positive vasculitides including:
  - Wegener's granulomatosis
  - microscopic polyarteritis
  - Churg–Strauss syndrome
- Anti-glomerular basement membrane (GBM) antibody disease
- Coeliac disease (gluten enteropathy)
- Primary biliary cirrhosis and autoimmune hepatitis
- Myasthenia gravis
- Idiopathic thrombocytopenic purpura (ITP) and haemolytic anaemia
- Thyrotoxicosis or hypothyroidism
- Addison's disease

unclear in many instances. Autoimmunity may be organ specific, as in autoimmune thyroid disease, or non-organ specific, when it is directed at self antigens that are not restricted to particular organs (Table 10.1). For example, some of the autoantibodies generated in systemic lupus erythematosus (SLE) bind DNA, histones, etc., and these antigens may be found in any injured tissue. Some autoantibodies are directly involved in disease pathogenesis. For example, the anti-neutrophil cyto-plasmic antigen autoantibody (ANCA) is undoubtedly involved in small vessel vasculitides, whereas the deposition of anti-glomerular basement membrane (GBM) antibody in the kidney is responsible for Goodpasture's disease. In contrast, the role of other autoantibodies such as rheumatoid factor or anti-nuclear antibodies (ANAs) in the disease process is much less clear. Despite these caveats, laboratory investiga-tions play an important role in the diagnosis of many conditions and in the monitoring of treatment. Immunologically based tests are also useful in non-autoimmune diseases affecting the haematopoietic or reticuloendothelial system, such as myeloma that is characterised by the production of a monoclonal paraprotein or excessive light chains.

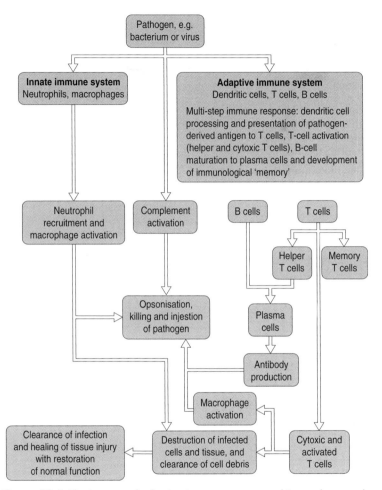

Figure 10.1 The innate and adaptive immune systems combine to detect and eliminate pathogenic organisms effectively.

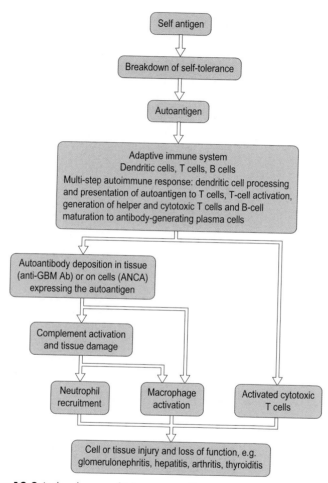

Figure 10.2 In the absence of tolerance to self antigens, the innate and adaptive immune systems may result in serious injury to and dysfunction of host tissues and organs.

Table 10.1 Autoantibodies and related conditions

Autoantibody	Associated conditions
Rheumatoid factor (0–20 IU/mL)	Present in about 80% of patients with rheumatoid arthritis
Antinuclear antibody (ANA)	SLE, though may be found in other conditions
Anti-double-stranded DNA antibodies (performed if ANA positive)	SLE
Anti-extractable nuclear antigen (ENA) – there are several antibodies in this category:	
• Anti-Ro	SLE, Sjögren's syndrome, systemic sclerosis
• Anti-La	Sjögren's syndrome, SLE
• Anti-Sm	SLE
• Anti-nRNP (nuclear ribonucleoproteins)	Mixed connective tissue disease
• Anti-Scl-70 (topoisomerase 1)	Systemic sclerosis
• Anti-centromere	Systemic sclerosis
• Anti-Jo-1	Dermatomyositis
Anti-neutrophil cytoplasmic antibody (ANCA)	Associated with small vessel vasculitides such as Wegener's granulomatosis (PR3 ANCA) and microscopic polyarteritis (MPO ANCA)
Anti-glomerular basement membrane antibody	Goodpasture's syndrome
Thyrotropin receptor antibodies (may be stimulatory or inhibitory)	Graves' disease (hyperthyroidism)
Anti-thyroglobulin and anti-thyroid peroxidase antibodies	Hashimoto's thyroiditis
Anti-gliadin antibody	Coeliac disease
Anti-endomysial antibody	
Anti-smooth muscle antibodies	Primary biliary cirrhosis and autoimmune hepatitis
Anti-mitochondrial antibodies	
Antibodies to the acetylcholine receptor	Myasthenia gravis
Anti-cardiolipin antibodies	Primary phospholipid syndrome, SLE
Anti-glutamic acid decarboxylase (GAD) antibody	May be found in patients with type 1 diabetes mellitus
Anti-islet cell antibody	
Anti-insulin antibody	

Autoantibodies

Circulating autoantibodies may be detected by immunofluorescence techniques using tissues or cells containing the target antigen. However, autoantibodies may also be detected by enzyme-linked immunosorbent assays (ELISAs) that use recombinant or purified antigens, if these are known. ANCAs may be divided into either proteinase 3 (PR3) ANCA or myeloperoxidase (MPO) ANCA, and separate ANCA ELISAs have been developed that use purified PR3 or MPO in order to detect autoantibodies that bind to particular neutrophil autoantigens. This is clinically helpful as the PR3 ANCA is characteristically present in Wegener's granulomatosis, whereas the MPO ANCA is typically found in microscopic polyarteritis and Churg–Strauss syndrome. Other techniques include immunodiffusion and particle agglutination (e.g. rheumatoid factor). Laboratories may offer several techniques for assessing individual autoantibodies such as ANCA (ELISA and immunofluorescence), and maximal diagnostic specificity is obtained by employing both techniques. In addition, the introduction of ELISA technology has also been informative as some patients exhibit ANCAs of unusual specificities. For example, occasional patients with inflammatory bowel disease or suppurative pulmonary disease such as bronchiectasis may develop antibodies directed against additional neutrophil antigens such as lactoferrin or elastase. These autoantibodies give a positive result in an immunfluoresence ANCA assay but are negative in specific PR3 or MPO ELISAs.

Rheumatoid factor is an IgM autoantibody directed at the Fc portion of immunoglobulin molecules and may thus form an immune complex with normal circulating immunoglobulin molecules. High titres of rheumatoid factor are found in approximately 80% of patients with rheumatoid arthritis, but patients may be negative early in the disease. A positive rheumatoid factor must be interpreted in the clinical context as it may be present in healthy elderly individuals and in patients with other connective tissue disorders such as Sjögren's syndrome and viral/bacterial infections. It is, however, of little use in monitoring the disease.

The measurement of anti-nuclear antibodies (ANAs) is a commonly used screening test for SLE. The ANA is also known as an anti-nuclear factor (ANF). Although a strongly positive ANA result is suggestive of SLE, this is also found in connective tissue diseases such as Sjögren's syndrome, rheumatoid arthritis, dermatomyositis, scleroderma, etc. Normal healthy individuals may also have a positive ANA finding.

If a patient has a significantly positive ANA, they should undergo testing for anti-double-stranded DNA antibodies, levels of which are typically raised in active SLE. Extractable nuclear antigens (ENAs) refer to antigens that are soluble in saline, and anti-ENA antibodies may be found in various conditions including SLE, Sjögren's syndrome, systemic sclerosis, CREST syndrome, mixed connective tissue disease and dermatomyositis (see Box 10.1).

Erythrocyte sedimentation rate (ESR)

A raised ESR is rather non-specific and this test is becoming performed less often. An increased ESR often reflects an acute-phase response such as a polyclonal increase in γ-globulins. The ESR is also raised in haematological conditions such as myeloma and Waldenström's macroglobulinaemia, as well as in connective tissue diseases such as temporal arteritis, polymyalgia rheumatica, etc.

C-reactive protein (CRP)

CRP is an acute-phase protein synthesised in the liver, and the production and release of CRP may be markedly increased in any condition associated with inflammation, e.g. infection, tissue injury, myocardial infarction. It is a sensitive indicator of sepsis and may be used to monitor the effectiveness of antibiotic therapy in acute infectious illnesses such as pneumonia, as well as infections requiring prolonged treatment such as infective endocarditis and osteomyelitis. CRP is also useful in the assessment and monitoring of immunological conditions such as rheumatoid arthritis, vasculitis, etc., and tends to reflect disease activity in the absence of infection.

Immunoglobulins and light chains

Measurement of serum immunoglobulins and immunoelectrophoresis is often performed in patients in whom a diagnosis of myeloma is suspected (Table 10.2). Patients with myeloma may exhibit a monoclonal paraprotein that represents the immunoglobulin generated by a malignant clone of plasma cells – the monoclonal nature of this immunoglobulin is proven by the demonstration of a single kappa (κ) or lambda (λ) specificity. A malignant paraprotein may be associated with an immune paresis characterised by diminished levels of the

---

Table 10.2 Common immunological screening investigations (note that units and normal ranges will vary between laboratories)

Investigation	Associated conditions
Complement assays: Total haemolytic complement (392–1019 U/mL) C3 (0.73–1.4 U/mL) C4 (0.12–0.3 U/mL)	Reduced complement activity and components may be found in conditions associated with increased complement turnover, e.g. active SLE, chronic infections such as endocarditis, etc. Patients may also exhibit isolated deficiencies in complement components
Immunoglobulin levels	Low levels of immunoglobulin may be found in patients with congenital or acquired immunoglobulin deficiencies as well as in patients with severe nephrotic syndrome. Immunoelectrophoresis can determine whether an increased immunoglobulin level is secondary to a polyclonal or monoclonal increase in immunoglobulins
IgG (6–15 g/L)	A polyclonal increase in IgG levels may be found in patients with acute or chronic inflammation or infection. A monoclonal increase in IgG may be seen in patients with myeloma (may be associated with an immune paresis) and benign monoclonal gammopathy (normal bone marrow examination)
IgM (0.35–0.9 g/L)	Increased in Waldenström's macroglobulinaemia (secondary to clonal proliferation of IgM-secreting plasma cells)
IgA (0.8–4.5 g/L)	May be increased in IgA nephropathy or liver disease

---

other immunoglobulins. The presence of free light chains in the urine or blood is also determined as part of a myeloma screen. It should be noted that some patients with myeloma do not have a circulating paraprotein, but show an excess of circulating or urinary light chains. Therefore both tests should be performed. A bone marrow examination is required to confirm a diagnosis of myeloma. Lastly, there are rare congenital conditions characterised by reduced levels of immunoglobulin production, e.g. Bruton's agammaglobulinaemia.

Complement

The complement system is composed of a large family of proteins and is an integral part of the innate immune system. There are three pathways within the complement system: the classical pathway, the alternative pathway and the mannose-binding lectin pathway. Activation of all three pathways results in the activation of a C3 convertase that converts C3 to C3b, which is deposited on the surface of microbes or cells. Further deposition of complement components results in the final assembly of the C5b-9 'membrane attack complex'. This complex forms a pore on the surface and results in cell lysis. Complement may be activated directly by microbes as well as immune complexes found in conditions such as SLE, cryoglobulinaemia and post-infectious glomerulonephritis. Such conditions may exhibit diminished complement levels when the disease is active and repeated measurement of complement levels is useful to monitor disease activity in SLE, etc. Excess complement consumption may also be found in chronic infections associated with immune complex formation, such as infective endocarditis. Patients may exhibit a genetic deficiency of complement components and it is interesting to note that patients with C3 deficiency have an increased incidence of SLE.

When should I consider performing immunological tests?

Consider performing immunological assays in:

1. All patients with symptoms affecting multiple systems. For example, young women with joint symptoms, a skin rash and haematuria/proteinuria may well have SLE, and measurement of ANA, anti-double-stranded DNA antibodies and complement is indicated. In addition, an ANCA assay should be considered in an elderly patient with haemoptysis, weight loss and a mass lesion on chest radiography, as Wegener's granulomatosis is part of the differential diagnosis.

2. All patients with an abnormal urinalysis and/or renal failure should undergo a comprehensive immunological assessment. Myeloma should be actively excluded in patients over the age of 40 years with renal impairment. Some assays such as those for ANCA or anti-GBM antibody will provide diagnostic information in patients with renal dysfunction.

3. Patients with symptoms suggesting immunodeficiency such as recurrent infections should be screened for an immunoglobulin or

complement deficiency. Patients with hypercalcaemia, anaemia, etc. should be screened for myeloma.

4. Patients with diseases affecting individual organs should be screened for the appropriate autoantibodies. For example, patients with liver disease should be screened for anti-smooth muscle, anti-mitochondrial and anti-microsomal antibodies, as these may be found in patients with primary biliary cirrhosis and autoimmune hepatitis. Testing for antibodies to the acetylcholine receptor should be considered in patients with muscular weakness suggestive of myasthenia gravis.

What do I do with the result?

Immunological tests are often used as screening tests in patients who are suspected of having an autoimmune or haematological condition. Negative investigations may allow the patient to be reassured. In contrast, positive test results reinforce the concern of significant underlying immunopathology. They may aid the diagnosis as in patients with vitamin B_{12} deficiency with positive autoantibodies to intrinsic factor. Positive tests may lead to further investigations that may be more specialised or invasive. For example, examination of the bone marrow may be required in patients in whom a monoclonal paraprotein or free urinary light chains were detected. Similarly, patients with evidence of renal dysfunction and a positive ANCA or active 'lupus serology' (positive ANA, raised titres of anti-double-stranded antibodies and hypocomplementaemia) require a renal biopsy to assess the level of renal inflammation, as this facilitates the formulation of a treatment strategy.

Immunological tests are also helpful in monitoring patients and tracking their response to treatment. Determination of CRP levels is very useful in patients with serious infection such as endocarditis or osteomyelitis, and a falling CRP concentration suggests effective anti-microbial treatment. Conversely, a failure of the CRP level to fall or an increasing CRP level would raise concerns about the efficacy of the antibiotic therapy (?antibiotic resistance) or the development of an abscess requiring radiological or surgical drainage. Paraprotein levels indicate the tumour burden in patients with myeloma, and should fall with treatment. Titres of ANCA and anti-GBM antibody are measured serially in patients with glomerulonephritis. A persistently positive ANCA indicates a higher potential for disease relapse, and also increases the risk of recurrent disease if a patient who has received a kidney transplant. In addition, the development of a positive ANCA in a previously ANCA-negative patient in clinical remission may herald a disease relapse; such patients require a careful assessment including analysis of urine by dipstick and microscopy, and investigation of renal function and CRP.

INDEX

Note: Page numbers in *italics* denote figures and tables